Written at Orford, Quebec

by

Kishori Aird, n.d.

Kishori Aird

DNA DEMYSTIFIED

VOLUME I

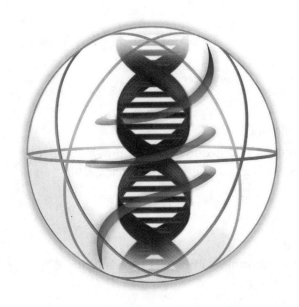

*A Practical Guide To Reprogramming
The 13 Helixes At Zero Point*

EDITOR: Copyright – © Kishori Institute, Inc.
P.O. Box 252
Magog, Quebec
JIX 3W8
Tel.: (819) 868-1284
Fax: (819) 868-9007
Web site: www.kishori.org

All rights reserved.

Assistant Editor: Jean Cloutier
Revision: Kim Bourgeois and Louise Drolet
Proofreading: Françoise McNeil
Graphics: Carl Lemyre
Layout: Rita Levig
Illustration: Devin Young
Translation: Les traductions Hi-trad. and Shawn Young

First Printing: November 2004

ISBN   2-9807441-2-3
Legal deposit – Bibliothèque nationale du Québec, 2004
Legal deposit – National Library of Canada, 2004

Distribution
United States
New Leaf Distributing Company, Lithia Springs, GA 301227-1557
1 800 326-2665
www.newleaf-dist.com/

Canada
Phoenix Distributors, Surrey, B.C.
1 800 563-6050
www.phoenixdistributors.biz/

Other: Bruno Simard
(819) 868-0595
Printed in Canada.

Author's Acknowledgements

I would like to thank my partner, Bruno Simard, whose support has kept me grounded and helped me have fun during this project. His spirituality, his affectionate support and his determination to be committed has made it possible for us to incorporate reprogramming DNA concepts into our daily lives.

I want to express my appreciation to my four Indigo children—Devin, Shawn, Marie-France and Merlin—who repeatedly aided and supported my work, simply by the spirit of their presence.

I want to express gratitude to my coach, Jean Cloutier, who was a constant source of encouragement and support. A master in the art of communication, he was able to share his knowledge and insights with me.

Special thanks to my friend Alice Melanson for her friendship and for the help she gave me in elaborating my ideas, which contributed immensely to the development of the protocols.

Thanks to everyone who read and revised the text and helped me make this happen.

A special thank you goes out to my students, who contributed greatly and participated in my training sessions, first on medical intuition and then, since the beginning of January 2000, in the reprogramming of DNA. They explored my ideas, put them into practice and, through numerous comments, helped me clarify my vision. They had the courage to say "yes" and to gain, one stage at a time, the control of their own genetic codes. It is a tremendous reward for an innovative person like myself to see my ideas integrated into everyday life. Finally, I would like to acknowledge all those who, directly or indirectly, were involved in the creation and distribution of this book.

Table of Contents

Introduction

It is easy these days to look at the world and think that we are living in chaotic times. It is surprising to realize to what extent old structures can adapt themselves in such turbulent period. Completely new concepts can be introduced into our collective thinking. Take as an example the twentieth century, especially the second half, which could not have been more chaotic, and think of what we take for granted. Then imagine what our ancestors would have thought of in-vitro fertilization and of the Internet to gain an understanding of how chaos can become a source of fascinating change.

We live in an era in which "truth" is being redefined. We are taught in all branches of science—especially in quantum physics—that solid matter no longer exists as we know it and that concrete reality is determined by our thoughts. From this we can conclude with certainty that the catastrophes we dread and that change our lives can also be an open door to new thoughts, behaviours and realities manifest. All we need to do is think back to the true story in the film *Lorenzo's Oil* to understand this fact. The parents, confronted with their son's presumably degenerative mental illness, refused to accept neither the medical prognosis nor social ostracism. Their rebellion, research and observation led them to new links and new connections in their way of thinking. This process resulted in the discovery of a cure. This story illustrates the course of almost all important human discoveries.

I am convinced that, because it is an invitation to redefine our reality, our current chaotic period represents an opportunity to reorganize and reprogram our DNA, our own genetic code.

The Power Over Our Reality

I decided to write this book now because I knew that the time had come to retake possession of ourselves. While scientists and pharmaceutical companies are trying to take over our genetic code by obtaining patents on our genes, we can regain the sovereignty of our own DNA—and therefore of our lives—and this power over our realities can, from now on, be encoded in our genes. If I had to summarize in one sentence the message that I wish to convey in this book, I would say: *"We have a lot more power than we think we do!"*

We already know that our attitude can influence our health and development. Several texts have has already been written on cellular reprogramming and on the psycho-neuro-immunology network. But, curiously enough, little documentation has been produced on DNA reprogramming other than incomplete information provided by scientists, and their partial knowledge on our DNA.

We use only a small percentage of our brain while awake! Our DNA does not operate at 100%! There is a multitude of possible combinations between the different inactive DNA proteins, to the extent that the biologists who have defined the human genome have concluded that 97% of our DNA is superfluous!!! Everything indicates that, as the human race mutated, a large part of our genetic heritage was lost. Several people even believe that, in the course of history, we have been subjected to genetic manipulations which have weakened our DNA.

In effect, it is as if we have an automobile equipped with all kinds of interesting options like electric windows and air conditioning, but that, for whatever reason, we do not use them. The salesperson did not inform us of all the vehicle's options, and for some unknown reason, we never even thought that those features were put in place for us to use. That is why I'm inviting you to make new links and ask yourself new questions regarding your genetic programs.

In order for us to gain a better understanding of the great leap which is currently taking place in the evolution of the human race, we have to understand the important role of the human genetic code in this evolution. DNA is very powerful and we need to own it back. Transgenic manipulations, governed by an industry that keeps the public in ignorance, clearly illustrate the issues.

I have been meditating for over thirty years and could sense in the course of those years of spiritual practice that a change in frequency was in fact occurring. I am convinced that the time has finally come to transform the old paradigms of our human genetic programs. The time has arrived when we can take back our collective heritage, a heritage we bear within, in the heart of every cell of our bodies. Moreover, everything indicates that our present planetary circumstances are conducive to reprogramming certain aspects of our junk or random DNA, that we can accomplish this on our own, and that the current activation of new helixes can accelerate this process of change.

The Genesis of this Book

The day I turned 40, I understood that, although I had accomplished everything that I wanted to do in my life, I had never lived in a permanent state of love. Therefore, as I prepared for the second part of my life, I pondered on this, and declared that I *chose* to live the half unfolding before me in a state of love, *even if* I did not know how. I wanted very much to discover what my life would be like in that state, so I summoned up all of my determination to persevere.

Since then, each time I have had to resolve problems, a fear or a doubt, I chose through my intention, to overcome it in a state of love, *even if* I absolutely had no idea how I was going to achieve that. When, like all mothers, I had to resolve conflicts, I *chose* to do it in a state of love, *even if* I did not know how. It was a personal choice, a way of life. At the time, I had no idea of the impact that this personal discipline would have on my work, which began two years later, on reprogramming the DNA.

In 1997, several months after the birth of my youngest son, I started my work on DNA. Three of us—all therapists—met once a month. We used imagination, medical intuition and visualization. One of us had been educated in medicine; the other had trained in metaphysics. As a naturopathic doctor and medical intuitive, I brought to the trio my experiences in alternative medicine.

From the very first meeting, we called upon the universal energy of the heart since I knew then that, irrevocably, we had to embark on this adventure in a state of love, and that exploring DNA outside of that frequency would have been impossible. In fact, all of the Reprogramming Protocols include verification in light of this energy.

We invested so much into this research that after two years the process had physically and mentally drained us to the point of wanting to abandon the whole project. At that point, we were not aware that experiments with new DNA helixes required greater vigilance in terms of our needs and physical abilities. We came to understand that we had to add another person to our team who would be able to keep us anchored. That is when my husband joined our team and took on the role of an anchor person to help us establish and maintain a sense of well being within our nervous, immune and endocrine systems while in the process of developing this project.

We were then able to resume our research. The more the frequency changed, the more we had to increase our levels of physical and spiritual resistance. We had to find a new method of working at an optimal pace without exceeding our limits. We met less often in order to take more time to integrate the data more fully.

When we had a sufficient amount of ideas and information to make the reprogramming of the DNA accessible and applicable in our daily lives, we decided to put an end to our group research. Our group dissolved, each of us keeping what we wanted from those years of research. As for me, I felt confident that I had collected enough information on DNA to incorporate the results of our research in both my daily life and in my teachings.

I must say that, throughout the process of developing the tools needed to reprogram DNA, I worked solely with people who were well grounded in their daily lives and who lived down-to-earth realities. I did not channel higher powers to obtain knowledge or to understand how to apply this knowledge to human biology. All members of our group, including myself, used intuition and imagination, in conjunction with our concrete knowledge acquired from our professional skills, to enter our bodies and take back the genetic code that lies dormant in our DNA. It is from my personal experience, my experimentations, my knowledge, as well as its synthesis and integration with the information I obtained from different sources, that I eventually developed an integrated knowledge of DNA.

In this respect, it can be said that this book is a compilation of my discoveries, thoughts and observations—including those of my students and our work group— as well as my conclusions and the treatments offered to my clients.

There is a forgotten force at the heart of DNA that allows us to shape our lives and identities. The more we know about DNA, the more we will become conscious of its value and the more we will gain respect vis-à-vis its codification and its power. The results obtained through experiments of this force are fascinating. My students, in DNA reprogramming, have attained an overall greater emotional maturity, more stable financial situations, clearer connections with their intuition and, most of all, the feeling of being in control of their destinies. They have gradually regained their power and integrated it into their daily lives. More importantly, their spirituality has stopped being trapped in an ethereal universe, disconnected from human life.

This is why I have chosen to end this introduction by quoting a client, Françoise L., who shared her experience in reprogramming her DNA:

When I ask myself what I gained from reprogramming my DNA, the first thing that comes to mind is that it gave me the opportunity to re-empower myself. The feeling of powerlessness that I had toward life in general is slowly disappearing. I now have a simple yet extraordinary tool that allows me to look inside myself in a profound way by identifying, among other things, programs that are no longer convenient for me and that I had no idea even existed. For example, I know more about (and in some cases I know with certainty) the origins of my fears. This allows me to integrate them so that I can continue to move forward in my life in a more confident way. I started reprogramming my DNA soon after a divorce. It was much easier to go through this painful experience that I had myself provoked. Reprogramming DNA helps one to communicate in a non-judgemental manner. My relationships with those close to me have improved and are so much more rewarding. I have a lot more confidence and, more importantly, I feel a sense of inner peace. I feel great and happy to be alive. I realize that the longer I stay in this state, the more I feel that I influence others around me. And that is exactly where the change is first felt: at the source. By changing oneself, we change the world! Is that not extraordinary?

Chapter 1

WE ARE PROGRAMMED

To fully grasp the importance of the information revealed in this book, an introduction to our genetic material must first be given. To learn how to use our DNA to improve our health, lives and evolution, we must remember that all of the commands and programs that manage our body and spirit are found within our DNA. DNA is what decides whether our eyes are going to be brown or blue, and whether our hair will be curly even if we would have preferred it to be straight! Therefore, we will begin by examining the nature and physical functions of our DNA from a scientific perspective before introducing its vibratory aspect.

The Physical Diagram of DNA

DNA (deoxyribonucleic acid) is found in the heart of each cell of our bodies. Inside the nucleus of each cell, DNA forms 46 distinct chromosomal strands (or chromosomes), which usually appear in the form of 23 pairs. Each chromosome is composed of multiple genes, which in turn are each responsible for either a function or a specific biological characteristic. To transmit its messages or instructions to the cells, DNA uses RNA (ribonucleic acid), which acts like a "telephone."

Moreover, DNA generates an electric current and, as a result, works like a small motor. Just as an electrical current travelling through a loop creates its own magnetic field, the DNA spiral, which curls back on itself, is sensitive to magnetic influences.

Another interesting DNA characteristic is that it emits light in the form of biophotons. This light, although extremely dim (its luminosity is equivalent to that of a candle seen from ten kilometres away), is highly consistent and regular, meaning that it works in phases, like lasers. In this manner, DNA is a kind of mini-laser. In fact, there is a possible link between consciousness and DNA's emission of photons. The splendid light which radiates from highly evolved people and saints could, in other words, be merely due to the activation of their DNA—a very fascinating concept indeed!

The best way to visualize the basic structure of our DNA is by first imagining a very long ladder with hundreds of thousands of steps. This ladder is "twisted" until its steps form a double spiral, otherwise known as a double helix. This double helix is also "twisted" and resembles a tangled-up telephone cord.

The ladder sides are chains of molecules of simple sugar and phosphate, and the steps are formed of four nucleic acids: adenine (A), thymine (T), cytosine (C) and guanine (G). To define DNA, we use four letters—A, T, C and G—or in other words, the first letter of each nucleic acid.

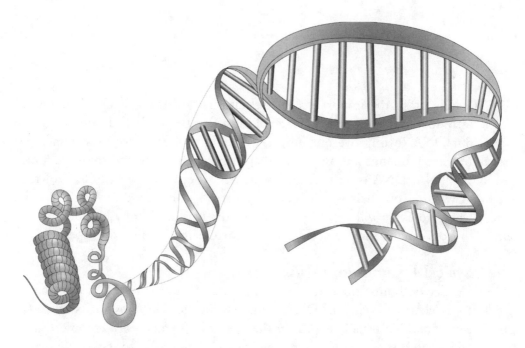

The four nucleic acids form pairs, and are organized in a set order: adenine (A) is always paired up with thymine (T) and together form either the AT or TA pair. Cytosine (C) is always paired up with guanine (G) to form the CG or GC pair. The nucleic acid pairs (AT or TA and CG or GC) then group into threes to form a coding unit called a **codon**. The "AT GC TA" chain, for example, constitutes a codon. Since nucleic acid pairs always gather in groups of three, there are 64 different possible combinations.

Codons themselves form a "code" or, more precisely, a **gene**. A gene can be made up of only a few codons or of several tens of thousands of them. In turn, genes group together to form a **chromosome**. A chromosome can include only a few genes or several thousand. Finally, the totality of all genes present in an organism, or the complete genetic code that sends out all the desired instructions to create and maintain all possible life, is called the **genome**.

DNA contains our ancestral and racial imprints, including codes that determine skin, hair and eye color, blood type, height and all other imaginable human traits. It creates different fingerprints for each person and is responsible for our strengths and natural abilities, as well as our hereditary diseases and congenital malformations. To realize the full potential of DNA, all you have to do is compare it to our super powerful computers, which function according to a binary system, alternating between only two numbers (or "letters")—0 and 1. Our DNA is even more powerful than these computers as it functions on a quaternary basis (the four letters A, T, G and C). In other words, gathered within the genetic material of each of our cells, is a database of extraordinary, almost unimaginable proportions.

On February 12, 2001, the international scientific community published the map of the human genome and announced that our genetic code included between 30,000 and 40,000 genes. However, this scientific data was—and still is—under evaluation and could change before a more "definitive" portrait of our genetic code is delivered. In fact, already in July of the same year, it was announced that there had been a misunderstanding and that we could now count between 50,000 and 100,000 genes in the human genetic code. This uncertainty could be explained by the enormity of the task at hand. Accurately defining the human genome could be compared to drawing up a topographical map which covers all the territory between New York and Los Angeles, including each and every little stream. Faced with this colossal job, the scientific community decided to proceed by offering a less detailed perspective. Rather than drawing such a detailed map, researchers aimed to produce something more equivalent to a satellite photo.

The "genome revolution" offers tremendous hope to victims of genetic diseases and, while the cartography of the genome is far from complete, it offers precious information on many levels. We now know that a chromosome can contain more than 5000 genes and that a single gene can contain dozens or even hundreds of thousands of codons. For example, a team of specialists from Toronto Hospital discovered a gene whose chemical composition, expressed as A, T, G and C (nucleic acids), is so long that, if it were printed, it would measure the length of a hospital's corridor. The lengthy dimension of this gene did not come as a surprise to the researchers, however. They think these codons make up the gene which contains the structure of the human brain. This gene could comprise one hundred thousand codons, or even more.

Junk or Random DNA

The dissemination of research results on the human genome reveals another fact that is pertinent to the topic of this book: biologists who have been working on the human genome have defined only 3% of our genetic code. Only three percent! According to scientists, some genetic combinations are active in our genetic code and others are latent. Our genetic heritage contains desert-like spaces between, and inside, our genes.

This means that scientists still do not know the purpose of 97% of our genetic code! This part of our DNA, which comprises only a few genes mainly grouped into "lots," is overlooked by scientists, who first baptized it as **junk or random DNA**, which basically means haphazard, rubbish or useless DNA. Remember that we are talking about 97% of our DNA! Then, it was re-baptized as *non-coding DNA*. Finally, since junk or random DNA does not produce protein, it was also named *non-protein DNA*. In other words, we know very little about this vast "desert-like territory" that constitutes 97% of our genetic code. For some scientists, these DNA strands seem to be illogical and do not provide any relevant information. For biologists, this part of our DNA could very well hold information on the origins of human life, including the secrets of our history.

For the time being, it is evident that the role played by junk or random DNA in our genetic programming remains a mystery to science. And yet this is precisely the territory we will focus on since **this latent part of our DNA is the one that could easily respond to intention and vibratory reprogramming**. However, before introducing the vibratory aspect of our DNA, it is important to mention two other pertinent scientific facts.

First of all, if you recall, four pairs of nucleic acids grouped in threes can supposedly form 64 combinations or codons. In reality, out of the 64 possible codons, there are only 20 that are active in humans (plus three others that serve as code switches or triggers). In other words, though invisible to the human eye, this minuscule biological diagram we call DNA determines all individual characteristics of every human being on Earth (everybody is unique) using less than half of the 64 possible combinations of the letters A, T, G and C of its "alphabet." It is like writing Shakespeare—or rather all of the literature ever written—with only ten letters of our alphabet. Where have all of the other combinations gone? Why are they not active? Science has not been able to answer this.

The other point that is important to mention here is that some children are currently coming into the world with a genetic code that is different from that of their elders. Dr. Berrenda Fox, from the Avalon Wellness Center located in Mount Shasta in California, has been able to show through blood tests that certain people have developed new helixes. In fact, she is currently working with three children who were born with a genetic code that includes three helixes rather than two, unlike their parents. These children are able to communicate with each other using telepathy and are gifted with exceptional psychic abilities. Dr. Fox believes that, on a scientific level, we could call this biological mutation. However, the scientific community refuses to talk about this in public for fear of alarming the public.

The Lost, Original DNA

A large part of human history remains a mystery despite all of the work done by our researchers and archaeologists. Is it not surprising that the history being taught in Western schools states that Antiquity only began in Egypt? We know practically nothing of Ancient China, the origins (or authors) of the Vedas in India, the Mayas and Incas, the Australian Aboriginals, the American Indians, or the peoples from the Pacific Islands. What about the dolmans of England, Peru's celestial landing grounds and the vanished civilizations like Atlantis and Lemuria? There are so many mysteries shrouded in our history. There are so many missing pieces to the puzzle that one can easily imagine that the same applies to the history of our genetics.

Throughout my life, I have lived in ashrams and have meditated up to five hours per day. But I always felt like I was going in circles. Then I worked non-stop to undo my childhood programming so that I could understand my built-in defence mechanisms. Despite all of that, I was aware of my tendency to keep taking the same route towards self-knowledge and I could not resign myself to the idea that we were forever condemned to "reinventing the wheel."

Then, in 1993, I read *Bringers of the Dawn: Teachings from the Pleiadians* by Barbara Marciniak. She was the first to mention the existence of ancient, unused genetic programs. She believed that the time had come for those programs to be reactivated on their own.

It was an original message, a previously unexplored avenue that offered a new perspective on the subject. It rang true for me that our genetic code had been manipulated, but that by reawakening our DNA in a state of love transcending duality, we could move forward. In fact, I had always thought that an extraordinary gift awaited us to compensate for the amount of courage it took to face the human experience. It is as if a part of me remembered a time in which we lived according to our full potential, guided from within by a highly functional genetic code.

I held this conviction even as a child. I remember an event that happened when I was in high school. My teacher insisted that happiness did not exist and I had a long discussion about the word "happiness" with her. I was 15 at the time and was convinced that if the word existed, then the state it described must have existed at some time in the past. At the time, I had no idea that I was going to set off on a long quest to prove my point, a quest that would lead me to the discovery of a perfect genetic program nestled within the mysterious folds of our vast unknown history, a program which seems to have been manipulated throughout the course of our evolution.

The Helixes of Our DNA

Various sources indicate that we have lost the original order of the divine plan within our DNA. I believe that the original DNA was perfectly suitable, powerful and functional. It contained the exact codes for ideal health, total adaptability and the state of contentment necessary for our incarnation here on Earth. Therefore, a large number of individuals interested in genetics believe that junk or random DNA contains the data of our genetic code's original plan before it was altered and underwent mutations. This has opened the door to much speculation.

The fact that children are currently being born with three helixes confirms Barbara Marciniak's theories and lends support to the multiple claims made by a large number of clairvoyants: our original DNA included a structure of at least 12 helixes rather than two, and the 10 lost helixes are currently being reactivated, if not physically, then at least vibrationally, in a growing percentage of the population.

As long as we have only two helixes (the physical ones), we will be limited and condemned to living in a world of duality. Yet, as you read on, you will discover that all is in place for us to activate, in a vibratory sense, the deactivated helixes of our DNA. I am convinced that within our junk or random DNA lies the memory of our deactivated helixes, and dispersed throughout, are the necessary codes to "reconnect them according to the original plan." Therefore, we must look beyond the set of references we currently possess regarding DNA and adhere to the principle that we can regroup, reactivate and reprogram our DNA/helixes OURSELVES. I also believe that, by reactivating the other helixes, we will finally be able to be OURSELVES, in all of our magnificence. Furthermore, I once read somewhere that, if only a small percentage of the world's population reactivated all of its helixes, the entire human race would reach higher levels of consciousness.

The 13th Helix

As I was saying, several sources lend support to the idea that the original configuration of our DNA included 12 helixes (see Appendix VIII). In the beginning, I based my work on this concept, and continued to do so up until December 31, 1999. That evening, three of us were meditating on the 13th chakra—the one that links us to darkness—when I discovered that there was also a 13th helix. This helix forms a sort of envelope, shaped like an "8", superimposed over the first 12 helixes (see diagram page 21).

Following this New Year's meditation session, I also understood that the 13th chakra/helix had neither form nor color (it was black), that it connected our being with a "neutral area" and that it circulated throughout all the other chakras and helixes. The role of the 13th helix is to anchor the reconnected helixes in the body, allowing energy to circulate freely between the 12 helixes, their chakras and the physical self.

By incorporating the 13th chakra/helix, it became very clear to me that we had to stop thinking in a binary way. Duality corresponds to an outdated vision, based on the first two helixes. When we reconnect all our helixes, and all 13 of them are activated (see Chapter 3), it becomes harder and harder to classify human experiences as either black or white, or good or bad. Our perception is no longer linear, but rather more circular or global.

Therefore, even if you have read many articles on the 12 helixes of our DNA, I invite you to modify your terminology and, from now on, incorporate the concept and amplitude of the 13th helix. In order to visualize the 12th and 13th helixes, you need to imagine a double spiral of DNA formed by two branches or physical helixes. Then imagine the DNA growing larger as ten other vibratory branches join the first two helixes (yet to be seen in a lab). Finally, imagine those 12 helixes completely enclosed in an envelope shaped like an "8," the 13th helix. You will then have the image of what DNA looks like with its 13 helixes. To help you visualize this, please examine the illustration below. You will also notice the link that exists between chakras and helixes.

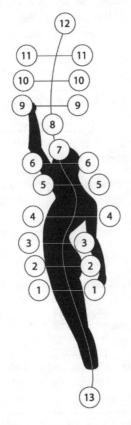

Diagram of the 13 chakras

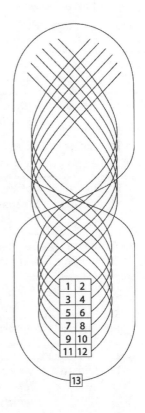

Diagram of the 12 helixes which are together and completely enclosed in an envelope shaped like an 8 by the 13th helix.

Now that we have touched lightly on the subject of the 13th helix, allow me to introduce how we define the 12 others. The definitions appearing in the table on the next page are not exhaustive. We are only beginning to rebuild our DNA, and I am convinced that we will have several other elements to add to this list in the next few years.

TABLE OF HELIXES

Helix 1	1st Chakra	*Physical and survival.*
Helix 2	2nd Chakra	*Physical, creativity, power and sexuality.*
Helix 3	3rd Chakra	*Clairvoyance (intuitive perception), power and will.*
Helix 4	4th Chakra	*Heart chakra, the center of compassion and feeling of complete connection with all things, the body's ability to vibrate to the frequency of the 13 helixes - electrical alignment.*
Helix 5	5th Chakra	*Speech, magnetic alignment – the body is aligned with its 13 helixes, creative freedom.*
Helix 6	6th Chakra	*Vision, subtle bodies – connection of the subtle bodies to the 13 helixes, discernment.*
Helix 7	7th Chakra	*Opens our awareness to the fact that our identity extends beyond the physical form – spirit/matter.*
Helix 8	8th Chakra	*Colors, connection with the entire world, original cause. This 8th chakra and the others that follow are found outside the physical body.*
Helix 9	9th Chakra	*Geometric forms of the universe – connection with the planets and asteroids – balance.*
Helix 10	10th Chakra	*Universal sounds, unions, connection with our universe and the solar system – unity.*
Helix 11	11th Chakra	*Interaction, inter-dimensional (multidimensional) – other universes (the void and the cosmic grid).*
Helix 12	12th Chakra	*To know irrevocably that we are human beings with a complete code – to feel fulfilled and at peace about our true identity, connection with the source.*
Helix 13	13th Chakra	*Anchors the reconnection in the physical body; allows energy to circulate freely between the 13 helixes and the body, thus cohabiting two spaces at a time, causing the terrestrial and celestial selves to merge.*

At the dawning of the 21st century, a time when we are discovering how easy it is to modify a genetic trait even before an embryo develops into a foetus, everything on our planet is conducive to our genetic reactivation. In fact, the power of the planet's electromagnetic field is constantly decreasing while the Earth's frequency is increasing. These earthly conditions are just right to increase the vibratory frequency of humans and, in doing so, will contribute to the activation of our original helixes.

These facts are nothing new. Many people on this planet, without having ever met each other, have made the same analysis and arrived at the same conclusions. For the first time in the history of human kind, we can speak the same fluid language, whose rules take into account the quantum concept stipulating that matter is not unchangeable.

Due to global changes such as electromagnetic forces and solar storms, we are currently experiencing a major turnaround, energetically speaking. This is the "chaos" that I referred to in the Introduction which will allow us to remodel our reality. It indicates that we currently possess the necessary information, understanding and confidence to carry out the task of reawakening our deactivated helixes, which lie dormant in our junk or random DNA along with the relics of our past programs. More importantly, it points to the fact that the reconnection of our 13 helixes and the activation of our junk or random DNA has already begun. It is a sign we have been awaiting for centuries. In other words, while we sit quietly in our suburban apartments thinking about more ordinary topics of interest, our helixes are being reconnected without our even being conscious of it. But I am getting ahead of myself here. We'll come back to this later. For now, there is one more thing I'd like to discuss before closing this chapter: the principle of the hundredth monkey and how it affects us.

The Hundredth Monkey

One of the aspects of my work on DNA which most excites me is that the reprogramming and restructuring we will launch, which involves consciously reawakening our helixes, will inevitably have an impact on humanity as a whole. All those who actively take part in repossessing their genetic code by reprogramming their DNA will directly contribute to the evolution of the human race.

In fact, by virtue of the hundredth monkey principle, each time someone reorganizes and reprograms a section of his or her DNA, this process benefits all of humanity. The hundredth monkey theory evolved from observing a colony of monkeys that lived on an island in Japan. In 1952, on the island of Koshima, scientists provided monkeys with sweet potatoes dropped in the sand. One day an adult female discovered that she could eat potatoes without the sand stuck to them by simply washing them in water. This female showed her new trick to her close friends and family, who, in turn, showed it to their own acquaintances until gradually, the whole colony had learned the "potato-washing technique." And then a strange phenomenon occurred. Let us say that 99 monkeys had learned this technique. Once the hundredth monkey had learned how to wash potatoes, all the rest of the monkeys on the island suddenly learned the technique as well. Moreover, scientists were surprised to see that monkeys from other colonies living far away on other islands, and even on other continents, were also washing their potatoes! The theory of the hundredth monkey was formulated to try to explain this phenomenon, which can be summarized in the following way: as soon as something new has been developed and integrated by a critical mass of subjects, this knowledge becomes accessible to the race as a whole.

In other words, each time a small part of the big picture is understood, it becomes available to the rest of the community, and there is no further need of pioneering work to access it. The hundredth monkey theory has also been used in trying to explain why important discoveries happen simultaneously in two separate areas without any contact between the inventors.

For us, the principle of the hundredth monkey means that anyone working on his or her DNA adds to the critical mass that will allow humanity as a whole to finally access the genetic codes which are hidden and scattered in junk or random DNA. Whenever people reprogram their genetic code, they automatically transmit the knowledge of this potential to others. When they reactivate lost programs, they become relay stations for their environment and energetically inform surrounding DNA of its potential for recoding. Each time one of us examines a section of our own DNA, asks the appropriate questions and puts order back into a specific area of our genetic code, this work becomes accessible to the entire community. He or she sends a new magnetic frequency out into the environment, informing others of the order of the process involved in reprogramming the genetic code. And so, the time will come when we too shall meet the threshold of the hundredth monkey. When that happens, humanity as a whole will receive this new information. What a grand day that will be!

This is how one person's work can move things forward for humanity—and this potential lies right here within us. The history of humankind includes many discoveries that have improved the quality of our lives through the extraordinary commitment of a small number of passionate people. But this time the discovery is major—fundamental—because it concerns all that determines our existence: DNA, our genetic program.

Consequently, even people who do not make a single effort to participate in this large restructuring will benefit from its effects. They are already being affected while they sit in front of their televisions, watching the daily news, wondering anxiously where the world is headed, while we—you and I — restructure ourselves, regaining our power and our sovereignty over our DNA. In doing so, we will feel the joy of consciously regaining possession of our divine heritage and will live a fascinating, fun and meaningful adventure.

Chapter 2

WE ARE THE PROGRAMMERS OF OUR DNA

Since DNA was discovered in the 1950s, scientists have convinced us that human beings were entirely determined by their genetic code and that there was nothing that we could do about it. Their stand was: we are programmed and genetic changes only evolve over long periods of time through slow processes. To this day, according to conventional science, the only way to alter our genetic code is to proceed mechanically (or in certain cases biochemically). In other words, take out a gene here, put one back there, destroy a few others with chemical products or viruses, etc.

Psychiatrists were the first to challenge the belief that it is impossible to influence our genetics through mind or spirit. Through observing individuals with "multiple personalities," they saw that each personality had its own name, vision of the world and way of relating to others (including sexually). However, let us remember that these different personalities all existed and alternated within the same body, causing physiological changes to occur within only minutes.

Of course, it is true that genetic programs do exist, determining our physical appearance, our biology, our innate abilities and even a considerable part of our psychology, including limitations over which we have no choice. What we are less certain of is that there is nothing we can do about it. We have a role to play. The scientific community does not have sole authority over the human genome.

By now, you have no doubt understood that if we imagine our junk or random DNA (that is 97% of our genes) and 41 out of 64 possible codons to be a restricted, futile and useless component of our DNA, then this is the idea that will resonate within us, shaping our reality. Conversely, if we are able to conceive of a greater reality, opening our minds to a larger temporal concept by remembering that junk or random DNA harnesses incredible power, our DNA's response will be boundless. It simply suffices to think of all that is possible with only 3% of our DNA in order to understand all the power that may exist in the remaining 97%.

Another challenge to the ivory tower of mechanistic science was imposed by quantum physics. According to the proponents of new physics, matter is not as "solid" as it appears; it is alterable, and it interacts with reality as well as with time. More specifically, when referring to the infinitesimal, quantum physicists have taught us that matter no longer has the same concrete reality: it is no longer matter but energy, and the form (concrete reality) it takes is influenced, and even determined, by the observer while obeying the laws of physics.

Scientists have even observed that DNA waves can be modified depending on the state of the observer's mind. For example, the spiral can shrivel up if we are in a state of weakness or depression, or become longer if we are in a state of creativity or happiness. This means that even the scientific world recognizes how our thoughts influence the physical conformation of DNA.

Nothing about this is imaginary. We have seen that DNA can be compared with a small electric motor, sensitive to magnetism. Clearly, this signifies that junk or random DNA can respond to our commands, choices and wishes, as well as to the quality of our energy. Consequently, all of our reprogramming work will be done on the vibratory level, targeting our junk or random DNA. Our tools will be **intention, kinesiology** (or another method of testing) and what I call the engineering of the **Reprogramming Protocols**. In the adventure that I am inviting you to embark upon, we will climb the steps one by one that will lead us to repossessing our potential and our genetic codes.

An intention is a command spoken out loud regarding the state in which we want to be. Stating an intention is a responsible action that allows individuals to regain control over their lives. Therefore, an intention is a sentence (a command) that states a new program to be installed within us and includes its unconscious, negative "by-default" counterpart. The first step to understanding and learning how to use intention is to leave behind wishful thinking and old programs which lead us to think that better times will come on their own. Instead, we must adopt the position of a programmer who knows how to use his or her doubts and weaknesses as the negative pole of a magnet, and perceive his or her active choices as the positive pole, in order to magnetize and command new possibilities. In reprogramming DNA, we will have to create new programs, and we shall do that through intention at the zero point of these two polarities.

Our Programs "By-Default"

Part of our DNA is made up of our original lost codes which are hidden somewhere in an unexplored zone that scientists call junk or random DNA; another part was programmed by our biological ancestors, through the generations; and yet another section was shaped by our parents and environment before we were old enough to have any choice in the matter. We were mostly subconsciously programmed by our earlier experiences. We tend to naturally go back to the latter, our unconscious "by-default" programs.

To explain what I mean when I refer to "by-default programming," allow me to use the analogy of computer operating systems, since DNA, including its operating systems, is made up of a series of programs.

Currently, 90% of personal computers run on an operating system called Windows, developed and marketed by Microsoft. Windows comes already installed on our computers when we purchase them and offers a series of amazing default options. This system has been working for so long that most of our correspondence via E-mail uses the same font. We even tend to think that a computer that does not display the Windows logo when we start it up is not real or good, and that it will not fully meet our needs. Since Windows is installed by default, and because its options or parameters are defined by default, many people are convinced that Windows is the only secure operating system compatible with our software. However, several years ago, other independent programmers decided to challenge Microsoft. They developed another operating system called Linux and offered it free of charge. Yet, Linux is not very popular. Even though Windows is often unstable, "bugged," complex and expensive, we tend to choose it by default. It is a little bit like our DNA: even though it's "bugged," we continue to choose its by-default programs.

When we were children, our environment "installed" in us programs that seemed as perfect as Windows since they were offered by a parental authority (Microsoft). Hence, our "by-default" programs are most often learned during childhood. For example, people who, as children, learned that to be loveable, they needed to be quiet and not make too much noise, will tend to automatically choose the "silent mode" whenever they need affection or tenderness. That is their "by-default" program. They buy Windows rather than Linux without even thinking. It is a by-default choice rather than a conscious one.

A child's brain and programs are easily influenced and manipulated (or programmable) since children tend to imitate their parents and their environment to feel a sense of belonging. This ability to imitate is what allows us, among other things, to learn our mother tongue. To be loved, we have all chosen programs, which, from a child's point of view, once seemed appropriate. The problem starts when we become adults since these deep-rooted and genetically-encoded programs are carried on by default.

To break away from our unconscious by-default programs, we must make conscious choices. That means working with conscious intentions rather than by-default intentions. A conscious intention is equivalent to clicking the control panel of our computer and choosing different settings from those installed by default. In other words, we must become similar to the independent programmers who created Linux and develop new programs in our DNA.

Wishful Thinking

Wishful thinking is one of the reasons we allow ourselves to be led by out-moded, by-default intentions. This expression refers to the habit we have of not paying attention to things, of not being bothered, of thinking that problems will sort themselves out in time. Wishful thinking is believing that one day everything will turn out okay without doing any inner work. That you will miraculously win a million dollars, or that all of a sudden the world will discover that you are a talented artist. In other words, it is believing that all of your wishes will come true as if by magic.

The first time I stopped to consider the meaning of the expression "wishful thinking" I really had to take an objective look at myself in order to fully comprehend how this concept applied to my own life. I realized that I had been hoping that, on some hypothetical day in the future, by sheer chemistry, I would have the life that would make me happy. I had not yet understood that I would have to stick to the task and come to terms with my vulnerabilities, rather than pushing them away, hoping that everything would resolve itself. I had many ups and downs before I was finally responsible enough to face up to the reality of my life.

From 1980 to 1990, wishful thinking frequently manifested in the form of affirmations. We thought that all we needed to do to improve our lives was to make positive statements, such as the classic, "Each day, I feel better and better." I used those affirmations often. However, I have to admit that they did not help me overcome the challenges that I had to deal with on a daily basis. Faced with the "catch-22" situations of everyday life and the constraints of the third dimension, affirmations seemed to create more frustration than contentment in my life. And yet, positive statements are intentions or commands in their own right, are they not?

Wishful thinking convinces us that everything should be simple, and consequently, we often get discouraged when it is not. It's at the root of the complaint we often hear in therapy, "Oh no, not that again! I thought I'd already dealt with that, that I was done with it."

When we hope to see our discomfort "magically" disappear, we abdicate our role as programmers, relinquishing our power over our reality. Nonetheless, life requires that we get involved in our evolution. It wants us to be imaginative co-creators who work with *conscious intention* while allowing our suffering the space it needs. It took several years for me to understand that by-default programs were cancelling the effect of my affirmations because I was in the habit of denying my pain and vulnerability, in other words, because I was denying my humanity and duality.

Vulnerability

To create an effective conscious intention, we first have to identify our pain and vulnerability, that is, the state in which we tend to slip back into our old programs, and then include these factors in our statement. Our contact with the divine, with our intuition and our DNA rests in our ability to read our discomfort and then simply install a new program using intention. Our vulnerability manifests itself in several ways. The following is a short list of some signs that indicate that we are in a vulnerable zone:

- Feeling stuck in one's personal development (due to a work group, a relationship, etc.);
- Feeling burdened by a sense of duty ("I have to…");
- Comparing oneself to others (feeling superior or inferior);
- Self-doubt ("What should I do? When should I do it? Where should I go?");
- Heart palpitations, shortness of breath, limiting physiological reactions;
- Obsessive speculation, the inability to let go;
- Lack of self-esteem ("I'm not nice," "I'm stupid," "I just can't do it.");
- Physical or emotional malaises that either pull you back into the past or propel you into the future;
- Any reaction or behaviour that is outdated, that is not grounded in current reality and that recurs unconsciously (being afraid of not satisfying clients, of appearing stupid, of being blamed even when you have done nothing wrong, etc.).

Past sufferings and joys cohabit inside of us. Both have their space and neither one should be eclipsed. What must end is not the suffering itself but rather the avoidance or rejection of suffering. Certain people believe that we need to avoid suffering by healing old programs, but in reality, accepting suffering is conducive to wholeness. All we need to do is give it some space and use it to make new choices. What we want to discard is the way in which vulnerability and past sufferings unconsciously control our present. In other words, we want to de-energize our by-default programs without ignoring the vulnerability and suffering responsible for their existence.

This is a very important point. In order to really create effective intentions that will act on our junk or random DNA, we need to be able to stay tuned to our vulnerable side. This implies that we also welcome and allow our vulnerability to remain present in our bodies rather than avoid it through mechanisms of denial. During difficult periods, we tend to dissociate ourselves from our bodies. We learned this mechanism of denial during childhood, the period when we were the least bonded to our physical selves and when it was easy to "leave the body." However, as adults, we cannot be open to our vulnerability if we are disconnected from our bodies.

To spend time with that vulnerable part of ourselves, that part that contains our sense of powerlessness, does not mean that our current reality will be permeated with a continuous sense of helplessness. It just means that we will be in contact with all aspects of ourselves and that we will need to work from the core of our beings to define the vision of our central intention. If I am not in contact with my vulnerable side, it will take control using by-default programs. If I *am* in contact with it, however, I will be the one who takes command, entering into a dialogue with it, thus redefining my reality. For example, I can say to my vulnerable side, "I will spend time with you, I will stay with you," while simultaneously saying, "*I choose* to live in a state of power *even if* a part of me is suffering." Simply stating an intention which includes my vulnerable side (*even if* there is a part of me that is suffering) gives me the right to choose a path other than the one that has been imposed on me by my by-default programs. I can now choose to live in a state of power. In other words, I am using my vulnerability to create rather than limit my potential. By doing so, it becomes an asset in my life.

To summarize, our "salvation," or our true power, comes from accepting our human nature as opposed to rejecting it. We tend to glorify our divinity by telling ourselves, "I'm only truly worthy when I'm living in the light." Real beauty and power, however, come from balancing our light and shadow, the latter being our more fragile, vulnerable side.

Recognizing Duality in Our Intentions

A magnet's effectiveness comes from the fact that it possesses two poles: one positive and one negative. The same goes for intentions or commands. For them to work, we need to consider both sides of the equation, including both poles of our duality. For example, "I choose to reconnect my 13 helixes" can only become a powerful intention if I add "*even if* I don't know how (or *even if* I feel powerless, etc.)." To include both poles will magnetize the conscious intention, thus making it effective and efficient.

Integrating duality into the formulation of my intention also allows me to ground it into my daily life. If I am able to endure an uncomfortable situation without wanting to make it go away, and if I am willing to tame it and explore it, I will then be equipped with the tools needed to use the emotion of vulnerability as the negative pole when formulating my intention. And I will do so without negative judgement. I am breaking away from a polarized way of thinking and entering a process that is no longer linear, but "circular" or global, and that goes hand in hand with the quantum dimension.

The following is another example of an intention that includes duality: "*Even though* I'm nervous because there is a dinner party for my uncle's birthday (negative polarity), *I choose* for things to be easy and to go smoothly (positive polarity)." Notice the usage of the terms "*I choose*" (positive polarity) and "*even though*" (negative polarity). This is how we build efficient conscious intentions. "*I choose... even though...*" are the key words in the technique of conscious intention. By using this formula, the intention "sticks" like a magnet to the refrigerator door. The statement following "*even though*" expresses vulnerability, the by-default program we wish to replace, while the statement that follows "*I choose*" expresses the new ₚ wish to install. If you adopt this method when formulating your intentioₙ sure to produce intentions which will work and have observable effects daily life.

This formula, in my opinion, is the only way to succeed in loving ourselves in the way we truly are. Evidently, it is difficult to love ourselves with all our vulnera-bilities, sufferings and weaknesses. However, it can be done with an intention, such as the following, which includes duality: "*I choose* to love myself *even if* I dislike the event which is taking place." That is why it is so important to stay in tune with our vulnerabilities and learn to use them to create a new reality for ourselves. If we take the time to clearly define the new program that we wish to install, we will learn to live with our darkness in a new paradigm which lies beyond the restrictions of the duality that has been imposed on us by our two physical helixes.

When I began using this technique, I started with small, simple things that I did frequently. For instance, while riding in my car, I would *choose* to believe that I would reach my destination feeling fresh and energized, *even* if the drive inconve-nienced me. I saw that things began to change for the better. Another simple exam-ple of this was the time I had to return a piece of clothing without the receipt. Before entering the store I simply stated my intention that the transaction go well *even if* I really did not believe it would. Amazingly, the salesperson granted my request without a problem! Another example is the time I woke up in the middle of a February night with the first signs of a cold. I immediately stated the following: "I *choose* to be healthy *even if* I don't have faith in my body." Suddenly, I had a high fever that lasted a few minutes, and then all of the symptoms disappeared. When, several weeks later, the symptoms returned, I *chose* to stop the flu again, using an intention, *even if* I did not believe I could do it twice in a row. It worked!

Through this process, I acquired greater self-confidence and stopped feeling helpless. My soul was reminded of its power and its ability to act despite the various challenges of life on this planet. And I understood that happiness and well-being result from conscious intentions.

If you lack confidence and have trouble formulating your own intentions, here are a few samples that were very useful for me. You can adapt them to your own sit-uation and make them your new by-default intentions:

- "I *choose* to love myself *even if* I don't."
- "I *choose* for this interview to be easy and effortless *even if* I've never done this before (or even if I've no experience in this field)."
- "I *choose* to be happy *even if* I don't know how."
- "I *choose* to have faith in my body *even if* I'm sick."
- "I *choose* to be competent *even if* I'm insecure."

The Feeling Is more Important than the Outcome

Intimate personal relationships are often very favourable environments in which to practise conscious intentions. Imagine this scenario: the partner of a very creative man has a by-default program that makes her feel inadequate each time he is in a highly creative state. Her feeling of inadequacy triggers a reaction in him, another unconscious by-default program that makes him feel guilty regarding his creative power. This also makes him feel uncomfortable and even aggressive around her. But rather than criticize his partner, which is not a good solution, he works with a conscious intention and says "*I choose*, while being in a state of creativity, to make everybody around me benefit *even if*, when I was a little boy, growing up in a big family, I had trouble asserting myself and remained soft-spoken and gentle." The problem disappeared! Similarly, if there is communication problem (or a separation), he can formulate an intention such as, "*I choose* to communicate easily and calmly when I'm in an intimate situation *even if* I don't know how (or *even if* I've trouble expressing myself because my father was so overbearing, etc.)."

Through stating intentions on a daily basis, I have learned two rules that I apply consistently to increase their effectiveness. The first one is that, once the intention is expressed, we must accept the way in which it manifests itself. Otherwise, we lose a lot of energy trying to control the result rather than welcoming the effect. Working on our general state of being rather than on specific preconceived results offers a new paradigm over and above the limitations imposed by our past experiences. It goes without saying that, while we describe the state in which we wish to live, it is okay to express our needs. Getting caught up in the details of the result is what we must learn to let go of. For example, if we wish to be in an intimate relationship, we could choose to attract someone who shares our frequency of energy (and whom we will not describe in minute detail!!!) *even if* we do not believe we can find such a person. We will then have to believe in the power of our intention. This magnetic power will attract the perfect match, although he or she may not necessarily be the type we had imagined.

Rather than saying "*I choose* to be in love with a rich, famous, beautiful person, etc. *even if* I've not met that person yet" (accent is on the specific form), it is best to say "*I choose* to live in a state of love, *even if* I'm obsessed with certain aspects of intimacy" (accent is on the general state of being). In the first case, we have more chances of failure, which may lead to depression or to feeling like a victim who is just plain unlucky. The second formulation, however, focuses more on the desired daily state of mind (the state of love). Everybody knows that when we lack self-love, we do not attract anyone. Conversely, several good matches often come into our lives once we've already fallen in love. This is simply because we are already in a loving "feeling" and have stopped searching for the specific "outcome."

Respect

The second rule that I have learned is that, in addition to including duality and emphasising one's general state of being rather than specific results, our intentions should be respectful of others. This is the reason an intention should never be directed toward a particular person. For example, instead of saying "I *choose* not to be affected by so and so *even if* I feel threatened by him/her," it is best to place the accent on a more general state of security: "*I choose* to feel secure, loved and respected *even though* I'm afraid."

This is the difference between establishing healthy boundaries and building walls to defend ourselves. If I state an intention aimed at a particular person, my stance is defensive and controlling. My intention is no longer pure and respectful of the free will of others. However, if my intention remains free of manipulativeness, and I establish a new program to replace an old one, I will then form new boundaries. These new boundaries are sound since they are of my own free will and consist of the new choices *I have made for myself*. If, on the contrary, I state an intention that is geared towards another person, I am defending myself from that person, implying right from the start that there is a reason to be defensive, which, may in fact, just be a false impression leftover from my by-default programs. Healthy boundaries established through pure intention are very solid, eliminating the need for defensiveness. Masters of martial arts provide a good example of how this works. True masters, for instance, rarely need to fight. They emanate such self-assurance, power and strength that others do not even dare challenge them.

As another example, one of my clients panicked just thinking about going to a family party. He feared that his presence was not really welcome since his mother had been ignoring him for several months and had rejected him. Intense scenes of rejection and confrontation kept racing through his mind. I helped him to form an intention based on his own state of being that did not involve his mother. He put forth a very simple intention, asking to be in a state of love during the gathering, *even if* he did not know how. And thanks to this intention, he was able to develop a new type of relationship with his mother. They were able to share a special moment in the "here and now" without interference from their old patterns. Upon his return, he was glowing with a new inner radiance. He was happy and peaceful without the attitude of one who has conquered. Over the years, I have noticed that repositioning conflicts through intention produces winners who shine without ego.

Imagine what can be achieved when intentions are used to directly reprogram DNA by creating new codes! My students, and those around me who are working in this field, have discovered that they can truly regain sovereignty over their DNA, and are surprised at the speed at which results can be obtained.

Now that we clearly understand the power of intention at zero point, a state which includes both polarities, we need to add another tool to be able to reprogram DNA: a method of communicating with our innate intelligence.

Kinesiology and Innate Intelligence

In 1992, I prayed to the God/Goddess of the body, that is, the form of divinity that manifests on the material plane as the physical self. Having meditated for 19 years, I felt that I was quite in touch with my spiritual, emotional and mental bodies. However, I knew practically nothing of my physical body. I was not sure why I was having an upset stomach or shoulder pain, and it seemed that all hypotheses were plausible. Therefore, I asked my body to break the silence. At first, I was convinced that it was through prayer, meditation and channelling that the answers would come to me. In other words, in a state reserved for the initiate. The problem, however, was that, in my humanness, I could not sit still during my meditation. Moreover, I was never able to get a clear picture of who I was praying to, and despite all of my attempts, had never been able to channel anyone other than myself.

And then, in answer to my prayers, I discovered kinesiology. Kinesiology made it very simple to establish contact with my body—my innate intelligence—and to receive answers that were as easy to understand as a simple "yes" or "no." To this day, I use this tool. Innate intelligence is the life force that makes the atom vibrate. In an atom, there is more space than matter, and it is in this space that innate intelligence resides. Innate intelligence is the part of me that can identify contaminated food when I do my grocery shopping, that tells me there are energetic distortions in my environment or that informs me that I have tapped into somebody else's emotions.

If originally you thought that I was the beholder of astonishing revelations, and that I could go deep inside myself through a special state of consciousness, I hope you now realize that this is not the case. Authors of esoteric books repeatedly state that while we tend to look outside ourselves for peace and contentment, we possess great wealth within, which we are able to access through a special state of consciousness. However, most often when I try to focus on my divine self, I end up thinking about mundane incidents that have recently happened to me.

My spiritual life is linked to the innate intelligence of my cells with which I communicate through kinesiology. Kinesiology allows me to chat daily with my innate intelligence. Isn't that wonderful? I am convinced that innate intelligence is our inner God/Goddess or, if you prefer, the Divine Self. However, for me, what really matters is not being part of some spiritual elite, but rather being able to function well in everyday life while communicating with my innate intelligence.

I truly use kinesiology for every purpose imaginable. For instance, I once found the perfect armchair for my living room only one hour before a reception I was hosting. I used kinesiology to give me clear directions and guide me through the city to the right store. I started by testing the different neighbourhoods of the city and then the streets of the selected neighbourhood. My tests indicated that the armchair I was looking for was in a store on Main Street. I found the store even though I had no prior notion of its existence. There was the exact armchair I needed! It was the right color and it was possible to have it delivered before the party. A girlfriend who was with me that day told me that this adventure had inspired her more than anything that I ever could have told her regarding innate intelligence.

I have so many other good stories concerning kinesiology! Take, for instance, the time I managed to reserve the perfect cottage on the American West Coast without ever having seen it, just by testing on the Internet. Of course, I also use kinesiology to find answers to less material concerns. For instance, I might test for the number of memories I have regarding a particular conflict. Or I might try to identify an emotion that has been encoded in me since the age of two regarding my sister.

As a medical intuitive, I establish contact with the body's innate intelligence through kinesiology. However, I do not test to know whether the muscular response is strong or weak as it is done in traditional kinesiology. I test muscular response to get a "yes" or "no" answer to my questions. If the muscular response is weak, I interpret it as a "yes"; if it is strong or resistant, I interpret it as a "no." I use this response as a positive or negative indicator, which gives me answers stemming from my innate intelligence. In other words, I have developed my own kinesiology technique and have baptized it "Reprogramming Kinesiology." I teach Medical Intuition and Reprogramming Kinesiology so that my students can learn to read and reprogram their health. They use this tool frequently because it allows them to easily communicate with their innate intelligence or their genetic code.

This method is what enables me to test questions and to come up with answers in the reprogramming of DNA. You too will need a method or a testing tool. If you want to learn about Reprogramming Kinesiology, you will find the necessary information in Appendix II. Otherwise, I invite you to use any tool that seems best suited to your needs to get "yes" or "no" answers to your questions. You could consider a pendulum, dreams, simple intuition, automatic writing or any other technique you find works for you. Just make sure that you are comfortable with whichever intuition tool you choose, and most importantly, select a method that offers clear, precise answers.

The Power in Asking the Right Questions

Innate intelligence contains a phenomenal amount of information and, since it functions in a non-linear way, it is easy to miss out on its treasures if you try to access it through linear thought. The power contained in asking the right questions is obvious when finding within ourselves the most valuable way of mastering our genetic code.

In all circumstances, the information received is directly related to the questions that we dare to ask. This is true scientifically, socially, spiritually, and in reprogramming DNA. In order to find the right answers, we must often ask questions which may initially seem unusual or ever preposterous. This is an essential condition to becoming a good DNA programmer. Here is an example of a question that I have asked myself: "Would my paternal diabetes gene, which causes my hypo-glycemia, accept to be modified? I received "yes" as an answer. Then I asked: "Can I make this genetic modification on a vibrational level?" and so on. By practising this technique, I discovered that I could quickly connect with my inner self simply by asking my innate intelligence increasingly unusual questions. For instance, I could ask: "Is there an emotion or a physical cause that prevents me from being able to meditate right now? And if so, which one?" Unconventional questions have allowed me to identify links that I would otherwise never have found and that have led me to a better understanding of my programs. This is where my strength lies since everything rests in the art of knowing how to ask these unconventional questions and the ability to trust the answers I receive. If you wish to learn about how to reprogram your DNA, then have fun asking yourself easy questions as well as other more complicated ones, like, for example, those related to reprogramming your DNA. You will discover a whole new wondrous world!

Reprogramming DNA

Mastering intention is essential to reclaiming your personal power. However, even after having worked on my by-default programs through conscious intention, it was still difficult to pick myself up and overcome inertia when I became paralysed by my emotions or my default programs. No matter how much I wanted to be happy and creative, I remained sensitive to foggy Monday mornings, heavy early-week traffic and the domestic requirements of my family life.

Yet, ever since I began using intention to restructure my DNA, I have felt a transformation occurring inside of me! I am still human, but I have changed so much that even Monday mornings are starting to look better!!! I finally have the feeling that my reality is changing, and the proof lies in the improvements taking place in my life on a very practical level. One thing is for sure: the more I get involved in my genetic code, the more I change. And the more I change, the more determined I am to install new paradigms in my reality, causing my family life to become more harmonious and my professional life more active.

The current planetary frequency resonates with acknowledging duality (as opposed to denying it) and installing the frequency of love within it. That is the new form of spirituality. It is one that involves creating a new frequency. The new paradigm to be installed involves integrating binary thought, assuming the zero point position, and accessing unconscious blockages in a spirit of kindness and acceptance. Our personal genetic manipulations will not be done in a laboratory. Reprogramming our junk or random DNA will be achieved by awakening to our role as programmers without judging our vulnerable side. Our tools will be inten-tion (including duality), our unconventional questions, our testing techniques (kinesiology, etc.), and the reprogramming protocols that I will be introducing in the next chapter.

In this way, by the power invested in us as human beings, we will reclaim the genetic wealth that is rightfully ours. We will seal our genetic programs through intention and we will declare before the universe that we have become the only decision-makers when it comes to our codification. We will remain the masters of our personal and human heritage.

I now invite you to be bold enough to explore these new frontiers. This is the real purpose of this book. We will also participate in defining and engineering our genetic codes, not in order to control others, or for the lure of gain, but to truly re-establish our original personal power. As far as I am concerned, this is our calling as human beings, even if everything is orchestrated in our collective unconscious to make us choose powerlessness over our role as programmers.

Moreover, choosing to become the programmer offers tremendous benefits. Increasing awareness of my ability to change, transform and take charge of my DNA gives me the sense that I am fully participating in creation rather than resigning myself to the role of an insignificant puppet. This makes me vibrate, and leaves me feeling free and peaceful. I no longer feel separated from the creative Source of the universe. I sense changes in a subtle, yet profoundly tangible way. When I undergo therapy or receive various treatments, for instance, I notice that my body is able to achieve a deeper state of regeneration. On a spiritual level, meditating becomes much easier. And finally, I am more prone to having metaphysical experiences.

Therefore, my main intention in this book is to share with all those who live with me here on Mother Earth the keys to unlocking the wealth of programs hidden in the center of our beings.

Chapter 3

REPROGRAMMING OUR DNA

Now that we have a better understanding of the scientific components of DNA, the role that consciousness plays in programming our genetic codes, and our responsibility as programmers, we will move on to the actual reprogramming. I have designed, tested and validated a series of protocols, which make up the present and following chapters. These protocols will allow you to reorganize and reprogram your genetic codes in order to regain sovereignty over your DNA.

If you have the impression that you need be extremely knowledgeable or spiritually evolved to re-code your personal genetic code, think again! When referring to DNA, we always imagine it as being a lot more complicated than it really is. The truth is that it is not necessary to be a clairvoyant, to be part of a select group of initiates or to even know the ABCs of telepathy to start reprogramming yourself. Since junk or random DNA has a vibratory, electromagnetic field that responds well to intention, this is the angle we will use to guide us as we do our reprogramming. And as we have already learned in the previous chapter, intention is both efficient and simple to use.

Formulating an intention is a process that is concise, easy to understand, and that triggers transformation. Changes tend to occur on an unconscious level, yet they provoke visible results. They manifest at different levels of our being, including our subtle bodies, our molecular structure, and even the space surrounding us. When reprogramming DNA, our goal is to use intention to install new programs or codes directly into our genes, targeting specific areas or "addresses." This process of reprogramming via intention is more detail-oriented than what we have seen in previous chapters, and requires that the programmer (you) proceed with utmost precision and great awareness. Having tested these requirements myself, I have developed a list of instructions that I have called *Reprogramming Protocols*.

I have invested many hours in developing these protocols since I do not practice channelling and did not want to base my work solely on images or visualization. My task consisted of "grasping" vibratory, ethereal concepts and translating them into an accessible and "earthly" language. I then created a system for my students that was both user-friendly and risk-free.

Each protocol is used to install a new program whose purpose could involve many things, including awakening dormant programs, eliminating faulty programs, repairing a faulty gene or replacing a by-default program. In other words, a protocol consists of a series of instructions to install a given program directly into our genes, delivering the new information to specific "addresses." Simply reading the protocols is liable to awaken or accelerate the re-connection of the helixes of your junk or random DNA in each of your cells. Furthermore, I know that many of you will sufficiently understand the essence of the protocols and processes to become autonomous in the reconstruction of your being through the genetic reprogramming of your current cellular programs.

Each protocol has been the object of long periods of testing. First, I tried them on myself, experimenting with the members of our initial small group of people. Then my students and clients tested them further. At each stage of the reprogramming process, I made sure that my protocols included instructions most conducive to awakening programs scattered throughout junk or random DNA. This book is the result of this lengthy task, but I only began writing it once I felt confident that we had achieved our goals: greater vitality, sharper intuition and a sense of freedom. I gave all that I could to the project because I felt that humanity needed to regain control of its DNA.

As you proceed, it is important to remember that the instructions which appear in the protocols have their *raison d'être* and have been established to guarantee safe DNA reprogramming. This is why I urge you to follow them to the letter, even if at times this may seem tedious or boring. I strongly suggest you do this at least until you have acquired enough experience to fully understand the validity of their order. You will know that you have truly mastered the reprogramming process of your DNA once you are able to intuit how the protocols were developed.

If, on the other hand, you find these protocols hermetic or incomprehensible, know that you can nonetheless use them just as efficiently as if you understood them intellectually. It is important not to get discouraged. Remember that your innate intelligence has access to all the information that comprises the collective unconscious. For the time being, your intellect is most likely just rebelling because it is not yet able to access this information consciously. It will eventually, though, so don't lose heart. Moreover, you may have an old by-default program that states that you are "incapable" of making the protocols work for you. If this is the case, use the intention "I can efficiently use these protocols *even if* I don't understand them" (or "*even if* I don't feel capable" or any other form of "*even if* I can't"). Gradually, as you keep using them, you will gain a greater understanding of the protocols and your positive results will be reassuring.

The Structure of the Protocols

As you will notice, each protocol has a three-stage structure:

First Stage: consists of verifying a series of points to be included in the reprogramming;

Second Stage: consists of commanding the installation of various aspects and ensures that the reprogramming occur at all desired levels;

Third Stage: consists of including any remaining data to ensure that the session is complete, closing the protocol and sealing the reprogramming.

Therefore, each step, numbered for more clarity, consists of a question to which the programmer must find an answer. (You can use kinesiology to do this or another testing tool of your choice.) The answer is, in itself, information that the innate intelligence will consider when installing the new program. Data can take many shapes and forms such as a confirmation that the new program is sealed or not sealed for example, or an insight and piece of information concerning a body part, an organ, an emotion, etc.

With the exception of the first two protocols, whose goal is to reconnect the helixes, all the protocols include an essential question, which constitutes, if you will, the pivotal moment of the reprogramming. It identifies the "genetic address" to which the new program will be delivered within the individual's junk or random DNA. How do we obtain this information? How do we know which chromosome is to receive the new program?

In reality, there are several ways to access our innate intelligence to obtain these answers. Some people visualize chromosomes 1 to 46, one at a time, and find the corresponding chromosome during their visualization process. They then repeat the process to find the gene and codon number. Others feel or see the answers by using a pendulum. What is important is that you have a precise tool that offers accurate answers. In fact, to reprogram DNA, you must be able to identify the exact chromosome (Nos. 1 to 46), gene (Nos. 1 to 5,000+), and number of codons (1 to 30,000+) into which the new program will be inserted. This is where I have found kinesiology to be very useful as it enables me to **find precise genetic addresses**, one of the key factors in reprogramming DNA. Other tools, however, can be used to obtain the same answers.

Each protocol is driven by an underlying basic intention that guides the reprogramming process as a whole. It is this intention that determines how the body's innate intelligence will use the data you gather as you move through the protocol. For example, the basic intention of all protocols is to reprogram DNA in an efficient and well-tolerated manner. Naturally, the fundamental intention of the protocol that serves to re-connect helixes is that the reconnection occur harmoniously and efficiently. The essential intention of the health-based protocol is to install the desired genetic code for health and longevity in the genes, and so on.

Since the protocols' verification process brings compiled data to a conscious level, the information is automatically recognized by the subject's innate intelligence and then included in the reprogramming based on the initial intention of the programmer. Suppose that you have "tested" that the program should be installed in Gene 536 of Chromosome 24. The programmer's conscious realization of this fact serves to install the data during the reprogramming session. However, this is only one piece of information needing to be processed. The others will be entered as you follow the remaining instructions of the protocol.

Due to the power of your basic intention, receiving answers that conflict with your goals should simply be viewed as information requiring adjustments by the body's innate intelligence. For example, imagine you are testing whether the new program is 100% sealed and you get a "NO" for an answer. That answer is data, an established fact. Since your original intention was that the program be 100% sealed, this piece of information is but a message sent to the innate intelligence. Based on this information, your innate intelligence will <u>automatically</u> adjust the reprogramming so that the new program is 100% sealed.

In other words, thanks to basic intention and innate intelligence, obtaining an answer contrary to the one you were hoping for is not an obstacle; it is a piece of data that becomes an instruction for innate intelligence, just like the commands included in the protocol. This combination of intention and innate intelligence is what allows us to use the protocols as a type of universal structure. The questions are the same for everyone, but the answers are unique to each person, meaning that the new programs can be fine-tuned and adjusted to suit the individual as you move through the protocols.

In short, the reprogramming process consists of commanding the installation of a new program on a specific gene located in a precise chromosome of the junk or random DNA. The precise genetic address to which the new program will be sent will be determined using kinesiology or another intuitive technique. Issued consciously, intention guides the reprogramming process because it is capable of influencing the arrangement of the information already inscribed in our genes.

DNA belongs to us and we can be its masters. Your genetic code belongs to you, and the time has come to fully repossess it. By becoming involved in reprogramming your DNA through the use of the protocols included in this book, you will begin to grasp the magnificence of human biological and spiritual functioning and you will become more aware of the very real possibility of being the true master of your DNA and its programs. You can also rid yourself of your by-default programs that you genetically inherited or that you have unconsciously acquired (patterns, habits, automatic defence mechanisms, faulty protein commands left behind by the flu virus or by chemical products, etc.).

Each protocol has a title and specific number to make it easy for you to refer to at any time. The current chapter includes the first 9 out of 17 protocols in the book. We will begin by working with Protocols 1, 2 and 3 as they form a series and are the basis of any subsequent work on reprogramming. Protocols 4 to 9 can be used in the order of your choice after you have completed the first three. However, before beginning Protocols 10 to 17, it is preferable to have worked on the first nine. For this reason, they have been placed in other chapters.

PROTOCOL NO. 1

Reconnecting the 12 Helixes

Up to about 20 years ago, most humans functioned with DNA made up of only two helixes. These are the ones visible through a microscope that scientists examine with the purpose of decoding the human genome. These helixes are connected and activated at conception. They guarantee the biological functions of our bodies and provide the required intelligence for our survival, reproduction and work.

However, for several years now, more and more people have had at least three or four connected helixes. These additional helixes provide better health, greater intuition and much more. They are usually vibratory, but as we saw in Chapter 1, in some cases, they can be physical. Scientists have observed that the DNA in certain children born over the last few years comprises three helixes that are visible through a microscope. In other words, we are currently experiencing a transformation of the human race and all we need to do is participate.

This is why Reprogramming Protocol 1 enables us to reconnect the ten missing helixes of our DNA. **Activating all 12 of your helixes, plus the 13th (Protocol 2), will open the door to the other protocols in the book.**

I suggest, as a first step in your apprenticeship as a "Genetic Programmer," that you simply read the first protocol. If the 12 helixes of your DNA are already connected (you can use kinesiology to find out if this is the case by asking, "Are my 12 helixes connected?") I strongly recommend that you read the protocol, nonetheless, as well as the detailed example that follows. This will help you to become familiar with the protocols since they are coded intuitively to awaken inner programs that have been dormant. Simply reading the protocols could trigger a conscious or unconscious reaction on a cellular level.

Obviously, reading the protocol will not automatically give you back your power as a "Genetic Programmer" all at once! The first protocol (and the others) could even seem obscure and complicated. Certain words and instructions may be a mystery to you and seem incongruous with your current knowledge. You may discover new notions and terms. In this case, I suggest that you refer to Appendix I for definitions.

It is also possible that you will understand Steps 1 to 7 of the protocol but find the 8th one incomprehensible. This is all very normal. Just remember, as I have already mentioned, that your innate intelligence has access to this information and it understands your intention. So don't worry, and trust that your innate intelligence will take care of what your intellect cannot yet grasp. Take your time reading the protocol. Let yourself be unconsciously drawn into this new way of working on yourself and follow this well-organized roadmap of protocols for your DNA. This first protocol will slowly sink in and help you understand the ones that follow. Get accustomed to them through reading.

Following Protocol 1 is a detailed example that will help you understand how to use it.

PROTOCOL NO. 1

Reconnecting the 12 Helixes

1st Stage of Protocol

1st Stage – PREPARATION

Identifies the object of the protocol as well as the data to be included in the reprogramming process.

Before beginning to test, set your intent by saying: ***I choose to be at zero point even if I don't know how.***

Use kinesiology (or another testing tool) to find the answers. Data thus obtained will be automatically processed by the body's innate intelligence and the genetic code's consciousness, in accordance with your intention.

The first two helixes (1 and 2) are always present. To know how to test a number, see Appendix II.

1. **TEST if all the helixes (3 to 12 inclusively) are reconnected.**
If YES, go directly to PROTOCOL No. 2.
If NO,
　　　A. **TEST which helix(es) is (are) already reconnected.**
　　　B. **TEST which helix(es) must be reconnected.**

We may get a NO for several reasons. We don't need to know why. Simply respect this information.

2. **TEST if it is appropriate to reconnect this (these) helix(es) now.**
If NO,
　　　DO NOT proceed with the reconnection now.
　　　TEST how much time is needed (days, weeks, months) before testing again.
If YES,

Commands should be spoken out loud.

　　　SAY: *I COMMAND the reconnection of helix No. ____ , (or of helixes Nos. ____ , ____ , etc.) and its (their) passage through the heart chakra.*

Some helixes may or may not need a color.

3. **TEST if it is necessary to install a color for each of the helixes.**
If YES,
　　　TEST which one for each helix.

Example: to install the 9ᵗʰ helix, install the 9ᵗʰ chakra. See the illustration on page 21.

4. **To reconnect helix(es) 8, 9, 10, 11 or 12,**
SAY: *I COMMAND that the chakra(s) corresponding to helix(es) No(s). ____ be installed.*

Test each element (helixes, etheric bodies and charkas) for each helix to be reconnected. If you get a NO, TEST which body or chakra (1 to 13).

5. TEST if the helix(es) is (are) connected in all of the chakras and etheric bodies.

See Table of Helixes on page 22. Read each definition while testing each word. The words that test YES are data, which will be taken into account when reprogramming.

6. TEST each word in the definition of each helix being reconnected.

The original DNA plan is the underlying diagram that precedes all genetic mutation. If this information still exists in a latent form, it will automatically be included in the reprogramming.

7. TEST if the program for connecting this (these) helix(es) already existed in the original divine plan of the person's DNA.
IF YES,
    A TEST if it can be reproduced here.
    B. TEST if a bridge must be installed.

A theme or another program may neutralize the installation of the new program.

8. TEST if there is a harmful program or theme in resonance (echo) or duality (polarity) that could interfere with the new program.

Memories of former programs are capable of interfering with the new program.

9. TEST if there are memories attached or linked to former programs that could interfere with reconnecting this (these) helix(es).
If YES, how many memories are there?

10. TEST if the reconnection could cause a disorder due to the electromagnetic field(s) of the helix(es), and if it must be readjusted to be tolerated.

The answer must be YES. If it isn't, incorporate the data in the reprogramming through intention.

11. TEST if the helix(es) is (are) at zero point.

Before installing the program, it may be necessary to enter other data.

12. TEST if it is necessary to enter other data in this program prior to its installation. If YES, go to Appendix III and follow the instructions to test which data must be entered in this reprogramming. Then, return to the protocol and proceed to the next stage.

2nd Stage – The installation takes into account all the data found in the first stage.

2nd Stage – INSTALLATION OF THE REPROGRAMMING

Insofar as the command is spoken out loud, each item is integrated in the reprogramming. Please use the tone of voice you would use for a prayer or hypnosis as the DNA responds to language spoken in this fashion.

1. SAY: *I COMMAND that the new helix(es) be installed in the nucleus of the master cell of the pineal gland in all lives and all dimensions.*

2. SAY: *I COMMAND that, from the pineal gland, this program reach:*
   A. *the endocrine glands;*
   B. *the brain, the nervous system and the peptides;*
   C. *the cells, the intra and extracellular fluids, the interstitial void, the atoms and the quantum elements (quarks, muons, strands,...);*
   D. *all of the helixes, chakras, etheric bodies, and the soul;*
   E. *another location* (see Appendix III).

If Point E tests YES, refer to Appendix III and find the area.

3. SAY: *I COMMAND the RNA to support and reconnect itself to this (these) new helix(es).*

49

The original DNA plan is the underlying pattern that precedes all genetic mutation.

4. **SAY: *I COMMAND* that helix(es) No(s). _____ return to the order of the perfect original program.**

5. **SAY: *I COMMAND* the speed of the photons and the structure of the DNA spiral to adjust themselves.**

6. **SAY: *I COMMAND* that the connection within the corpus callosum of the brain be restored according to the original divine plan.**

The telomere is part of the very structure of the chromosome. It is a protein found at the ends of the chromosomal strands in DNA that protects these strands. In simpler terms, it is the end of each chromosome. The telomerase is an enzyme that acts as the "glue" of the telomere.

7. **SAY: *I COMMAND* the perfect integrity of the telomere and the telomerase.**

Refer to Appendex VII for a list of systems.

8. **SAY: *I COMMAND* that any residues from old programs be eliminated through the appropriate systems.**

9. **SAY: *I COMMAND* that the helix(es) be perfectly sealed.**

Refer to Appendix I for the definition of Merkabah.

10. **SAY: *I COMMAND* that the Merkabah be perfectly sealed.**

11. **SAY: *I COMMAND* that no radiation affect the DNA or RNA.**

12. **SAY: *I COMMAND* that the helix(es) be reconnected until further notice, in the brain stem, here and now.**

13. **SAY:** *I COMMAND that the reconnection of this (these) new helix(es) be perfectly tolerated and integrated and that this occurs at zero point.*

ESSENTIAL POINT
in reprogramming

14. **SAY:** *I COMMAND that the power, the harmony and the purity of this (these) new helix(es) be installed in the DNA and be perfectly activated.*

3rd Stage

3rd Stage – CONCLUSION OF THE PROTOCOL

The installation of other data may be required before concluding the protocol.

15. **TEST if it is necessary to include other data in the reprogramming for it to be effective, tolerated or integrated.** If YES, go to Appendix III and follow the instructions to test which data must be entered in this reprogramming. Then, return to the protocol and proceed to Step 16.

This closes the protocol.

16. **SAY:** *I COMMAND that this reprogramming be tolerated and integrated, according to the original divine plan, in the frequency of love, even if our helixes have been deactivated in the past.*

This seals the reprogramming.

17. **SAY:** *I COMMAND that this regeneration be complete and sealed, until further notice from ... (the person being reprogrammed).*

Procedure for Protocol 1

The protocols are a universal structure permitting us to find data unique to every person. To create usable and simple protocols that allow us to tap into all possibilities, I constructed them so that you could access all sorts of data that would have been impossible to include in each one. This is why there are two steps in every protocol—at the end of stage 1 (Preparation) and during stage 3, just before closing the protocol (Conclusion)—where you must verify if other data from Appendix III need to be included for the reprogramming to be effective. This "other data" can be of any nature because it is unique to each individual's history and biology.

Of course, it is impossible to include in this book all conceivable data. However, it is possible to establish a flexible framework within which one can successfully pinpoint an impressive amount of precise and applicable data. This is how I prepared Appendixes III, IV, V, VI and VII. These appendixes comprise both specific data and categories of data that will open the door to an infinite number of possibilities. When additional data is required, the protocols will generally refer you to Appendix III, which comprises the key to the other appendixes.

As you browse the detailed example of Protocol 1, keep in mind that when you try it out, you will obtain answers by testing each item using kinesiology or another tool. Your innate intelligence will process the data you come up with or make appropriate adjustments according to your intention. Thus, every datum will act like an intention and trigger the reorganization of your genetic programming within your junk or random DNA, which will record this command on a vibratory level.

Russian scientists have discovered that DNA can respond to language, especially to the tone of voice used when praying or inducing hypnosis. This explains why we verbalize the commands we want to include in the reprogramming protocol when we reach the second and third stages.

Protocol No. 1: a Detailed Example

We will work with the following example to help us understand how to use Protocol No. 1 as well as the other protocols in the book.

1st Stage – PREPARATION

Use kinesiology (or another testing tool) to find the answers. Data thus obtained will be automatically processed by the body's innate intelligence and the genetic code's consciousness, in accordance with your intention.

This means, for example, that if we test the level of integrity and obtain a percentage lower than 100%, or when it is necessary to get a YES answer and we get a NO (or vice versa), this data should be viewed as facts that will **automatically** be adjusted by the reprogramming process. In other words, it is not necessary to address the result directly or try to "treat" it. Innate intelligence will include it as a "fact."

When teaching, students frequently asked what to do with the items that do not test. **Data thus obtained has been identified by the innate intelligence and will be included automatically in the new program.**

Purpose of the Protocol
My client asks me to verify if his/her helixes are all reconnected and, if possible, to reconnect those that are not. My intention is that this be done in such a manner that the reconnection be perfectly tolerated and integrated at zero point. I use kinesiology to find the answers.

1. **TEST if all the helixes (3 to 12 inclusively) are reconnected. If YES, go to PRO-TOCOL No. 2.**
   I get a NO.
   If NO,
   a) TEST which helix(es) is (are) already reconnected.
   a) To test, I ask the question: Is helix 3 (then 4, 5, and so on until 12) reconnected? And I note all those that test NO – in this case, the 6th, 10th and 12th.
   b) TEST which helix(es) must be reconnected.
   b) I test with the following question: Can I install these three helixes at the same time? I get a NO.
   Hence, I test the three helixes (6th, 10th and 12th), asking the question: Can I install the 6th (then the 10th, then the 12th) in this reprogramming? I get a YES for helixes 6 and 12. Using intention, I include these two helixes in the reprogramming and note that it will be necessary to do another reprogramming with this protocol at another time to install the 10th helix.

2. **TEST if it is appropriate to reconnect this (these) helix(es) now.**

   To TEST, I ask the question: Is it appropriate at this time to reconnect helixes 6 and 12 for this person?

   If NO,

   DO NOT proceed with the reconnection now.

   TEST how much time is needed (days, weeks, months) before testing again.

   I get a YES.

   If YES,

   SAY: *I COMMAND the reconnection of helix No. ____, (or of helixes Nos. ____, ____, etc.) and its (their) passage through the heart chakra.*

   I say out loud: I command the reconnection of helixes 6 and 12 and their passage through the heart chakra.

3. **TEST if it is necessary to install a color for each of the helixes.**

   If YES,

   TEST which one for each helix.

   I must install a color for the 6th helix. I test a series of colors and get a YES for violet. This information registers itself automatically through intent.

   For the 12th helix, I got a NO.

4. **To reconnect helix(es) 8, 9, 10, 11 or 12,**

   SAY: *I COMMAND that the chakra(s) corresponding to helix No(s). ____ be installed.*

   As I am installing the 12th helix, I say out loud: I command that the chakra corresponding to the 12th helix be installed.

5. **TEST if the helix(es) is (are) connected to all of the chakras and etheric bodies.**

   The 12th helix is not circulating in all the etheric bodies. I test in which body it is not circulating, and get the 3rd and 5th bodies. This information registers automatically in the reprogramming through intent.

6. **TEST each word in the definition of each helix being reconnected.**

   I refer to the "Table of Helixes" on page 22. I read the definition of the 6th helix while testing each word. The words "subtle body" and "discernment" test. For the 12th helix, only the word "identity" does test.

   I know that this data is now registered in the reprogramming.

7. **TEST if the program for connecting this (these) helix(es) already existed in the original divine plan of the person's DNA.**

   There are many programs that could have once existed in the original divine plan but have since been disconnected. They are still present and available in DNA.

If YES,
A. TEST if it can be reproduced here.
A. I get a YES.
B. TEST if a bridge must be installed.
B. I also get a YES. This data will be automatically included.

8. **TEST if there is a harmful program or theme in resonance (echo) or duality (polarity) that could interfere with the new program.**
   I test each word of the sentence and get a NO for the words "program," "harmful" and "polarity," as well as for the rest of the sentence, that is, "that could interfere with the new program." I know that this information is automatically registered in the reprogramming as a function of my basic intent, so I go on to the next step.

9. **TEST if there are memories attached or linked to former programs that could interfere with reconnecting this (these) helix(es).**
   By testing each word as I read, I discover that there are indeed attached memories.
   If YES, how many memories are there?
   There are three.

10. **TEST if the reconnection could cause a disorder due to the electromagnetic field(s) of the helix(es), and if it must be readjusted to be tolerated.**
    I test this for both helixes. There is nothing that tests for helix 6, but I get a YES for the 12th helix and my intent is that it be automatically readjusted.

11. **TEST if the helix(es) is (are) at zero point.**
    Only the 12th helix is not at zero point. Of course my intent is that it be brought back to zero point through reprogramming.

12. **TEST if it is necessary to enter other data in this program prior to its installation.** If YES, go to Appendix III and follow the instructions to test which data must be entered in this reprogramming. Then, return to the protocol and proceed to the next stage.
    I get a YES and go to Appendix III to find what it is.
    I first test how many items I need here, and get two.
    By testing in Appendix III, I first find an emotion (element No. 1 of Appendix III). To determine which one it is, I go to Appendix IV where I find the emotion "sitting on the fence." I thus have my first piece of information.
    I return to Appendix III to find the second piece of data, and I get "Virus" (No. 5).
    Since these two items are now entered in the reprogramming, I can proceed with the installation.

2nd Stage — INSTALLATION OF THE REPROGRAMMING

WHEN WE REACH THE 2nd STAGE IN ALL OF THE PROTOCOLS, EVERY STEP takes the form of a COMMAND, so we do not need to use kinesiology or any other testing methods. As we have already expressed the intention to be at zero point at the beginning of the protocol, we do not need to reaffirm it. According to some Russian researchers, the DNA responds to A TONE OF VOICE SIMILAR TO THE ONE USED WHEN PRAYING OR WHEN INDUCING A HYPNOTIC TRANCE. Make sure that you speak the commands out loud using that tone of voice.

1. **SAY: *I COMMAND that the new helix(es) be installed in the nucleus of the master cell of the pineal gland in all lives and all dimensions.***
   I say out loud "I command that the new helixes be installed in the nucleus of the master cell of the pineal gland in all lives and in all dimensions."

2. **SAY: *I COMMAND that, from the pineal gland, this program reach:***
   A. *the endocrine glands;*
   B. *the brain, the nervous system and the peptides;*
   C. *the cells, the intra and extracellular fluids, the interstitial void, the atoms and the quantum elements (quarks, muons, strands, etc.);*
   D. *all of the helixes, chakras, etheric bodies, and the soul;*
   E. *another location* (see Appendix III).
   I must test item E and if I get a YES, I test to see if it is the 6th helix or the 12th helix, which is affected, or if it is both. I find that it is both. So I go to Appendix III, item 16. I get "spleen" for the 6th helix and "liver" for the 12th. I therefore energetically enter these data in the reprogramming.
   Strands, quarks and muons are infinitely small parts of the atom, that is to say quantum parts.

3. **SAY: *I COMMAND the RNA to support and reconnect itself to this (these) new helix(es).***
   The RNA must carry the information which is delivered by the DNA, but it must also support it because it is equipped with an "interference" program which allows it to cancel the commands of certain genes.

4. **SAY: *I COMMAND that helix(es) No(s). ____ return(s) to the order of the perfect original program.***
   Say the command out loud as if you were saying a prayer.

5. **SAY: *I COMMAND the speed of the photons and the structure of the DNA spiral to adjust themselves.***
    Go to Chapter I for the definition of the photons.

6. **SAY: *I COMMAND that the connection within the corpus callosum of the brain be restored according to the original divine plan.***
    This data will be automatically registered in the program.

7. **SAY: *I COMMAND the perfect integrity of the telomere and the telomerase.***
    The telomere is part of the very structure of the chromosome. It is a protein found at the end of the chromosomal strands in the DNA that serves to protect these strands when they copy themselves. The telomerase is an enzyme that acts as the "glue" of the telomere.

8. **SAY: *I COMMAND that the residues from old programs be eliminated through the appropriate systems.***
    You will find a list of the systems in Appendix VII.

9. **SAY: *I COMMAND that the helix(es) be perfectly sealed.***
    This means ordering that the 6th and the 12th helixes be perfectly sealed.

10. **SAY: *I COMMAND that the Merkabah be perfectly sealed.***
    The Merkabah, which is an energetic field, has to be completely sealed. (See the Lexicon in Appendix I.)

11. **SAY: *I COMMAND that no radiation affect the DNA or RNA.***
    Radiation can act like a toxin. By this command and the two before, I make sure that the genetic code and the Merkabah are sealed and protected.

12. **SAY: *I COMMAND that the helix(es) be reconnected until further notice, in the brain stem, here and now.***
    Say the command out loud as if you were saying a prayer.

13. **SAY: *I COMMAND that the reconnection of this (these) new helix(es) be perfectly tolerated and integrated and that this occurs at zero point.***
    This means that the reconnection of both helixes is perfectly tolerated and integrated at zero point. This will prevent further irritation of the person's nervous system.

14. **SAY: *I COMMAND that the power, harmony and purity of this (these) new helix(es) be installed in the DNA and be perfectly activated.***
    I say this sentence out loud so that the information will be included in the reprogramming in such a way that the innate intelligence will make the necessary adjustments.

3rd Stage – CONCLUSION OF THE PROTOCOL

15.TEST if it is necessary to include other data in the reprogramming for it to be effective, tolerated or integrated.

If YES, go to Appendix III and follow the instructions to test which data must be entered in this reprogramming. Then, return to the protocol and proceed to Step 16.

I get a YES. Now that I have entered all the preceding data in the reprogramming, I go to Appendix III to see which elements I must enter to end this session:

I first test how many items I need and obtain three. The first is a shock at age 4 (No. 19). The second concerns chemical products (No. 6). The third concerns the liver (No. 17). I do not need to search any further because the innate intelligence knows of the shock in question, the chemical product at hand, and the present state of the liver. I therefore go to the next step.

16.SAY: *I COMMAND* that this reprogramming be tolerated and integrated, according to the original divine plan, in the frequency of love, even if our helixes have been deactivated in the past.

I end the reprogramming with this command spoken out loud.

17.SAY: *I COMMAND* that this regeneration be complete and sealed, until further notice, from ...(the person being reprogrammed).

I seal the reprogramming with this command, in such a way that nothing or no one can alter the DNA of the person being reprogrammed except himself/herself at his/her request.

Installing and Reconnecting the 13th Helix

On the path towards regaining sovereignty over our DNA, Protocol No. 2 was designed to permit the reconnection of the 13th helix and its corresponding chakra. Make sure, before using this protocol, that your first 12 helixes are reconnected.

To access the 13th helix, it is necessary to have installed the 10 other lost helixes. In other words, you need to have completed Protocol 1 so that you have 12 active helixes with which you are in contact. The 13th helix, and its associated 13th chakra, circulate through all other helixes and their chakras. Consequently, we can make the energy circulate freely between the 13 helixes and the physical body. This brings us beyond a state of duality since the 13th chakra unites shadow and light and grounds this union on the physical plane.

This is known as the bridge between Worlds, the point of equilibrium I refer to as "zero point" throughout this book. Accessible via the 13th helix, it is through this zero point that Masters are able to enter and exit the worlds. They succeed by merging their terrestrial and celestial selves, occupying two spaces at the same time.

PROTOCOL NO. 2

Installing and Reconnecting the 13th Helix

1st Stage of Protocol

1st Stage – PREPARATION

Identifies the object of the protocol as well as the data to be included in the reprogramming process.

Before beginning to test, set your intent by saying: *I choose to be at zero point even if I don't know how.*

Use kinesiology (or another testing tool) to find the answers. Data thus obtained will be automatically processed by the body's innate intelligence and the genetic code's conscious- ness, in accordance with your intention.

The first two helixes (1 and 2) are always present.

1. **A. First TEST if the 12 helixes are reconnected.**
       If NO, go to Protocol No. 1.
    B. TEST if the 13th helix is already reconnected.
       If YES, go to Protocol No. 3.
       If NO, go to Step 2.

We may obtain a NO for several reasons. We don't need to know why. Simply respect this information.

2. **TEST if it is appropriate to reconnect the 13th helix now.**
    If NO,
        DO NOT proceed with the reconnection now.
        TEST how much time is needed (days, weeks, months) before re-testing if it is appropriate to reconnect.
    If YES,

Commands should be spoken out loud.

        SAY: I COMMAND that the 13th helix and its program be installed in the body, pass by the heart chakra and move up the body, forming a figure 8.
        (See the diagram on page 21.)

By this command, colors black and white do not mix (which would give gray).

3. **SAY: I COMMAND the cohabitation of the colors black and white.**

Refer to the table on page 22 to get a better picture of the 13 chakras.

4. **SAY: I COMMAND the installation of the 13th chakra, for the reconnection between sky and earth.**

See Table of Helixes on page 22. Read the definition while testing each word. The words which test YES are the data required for the reprogramming.

5. TEST each word in the definition of the 13th helix.

The original DNA plan is the underlying diagram that precedes all genetic mutation. If this information still exists in a latent form, it will automatically be included in the reprogramming.

6. TEST if the reconnection program of the 13th helix once existed in the original divine plan of the person's DNA. If YES,
　　A. TEST if it can be reproduced here.
　　B. TEST if a bridge must be installed.

A theme or another program may neutralize the installation of the new program.

7. TEST if there is a harmful program or theme in resonance (echo) or duality (polarity) that could interfere with the new program.

Memories of former programs are capable of interfering with the new program.

8. TEST if there are memories attached or linked to former programs that could interfere with the reconnection of the 13th helix.
If YES, how many memories are there?

Each time we test something, the data obtained is integrated automatically in the reprogramming.

9. TEST if the 13th helix circulates through all chakras, etheric bodies and helixes.

10. TEST if the person is connected to the energy filaments of light and darkness at zero point.

Reconnecting the 13th helix allows the two polarities to coexist without cancelling each other out — rather than existing in a state of opposition or polarization.

11. TEST to ensure that the person can maintain light and darkness simultaneously without their cancelling each other out in the 13 helixes, all the chakras and etheric bodies, and the soul.

Commands should be spoken out loud. Use the tone of voice you would use for a prayer or hypnosis.

12. SAY: *I COMMAND* that the galactic body be anchored to the physical body on Earth through the 13th helix.

13. TEST to determine if the person is connected to his/her galactic vehicle.

The answer must be YES. If it isn't, this data will automatically be included in the reprogramming.

14. TEST to make sure that the connection between the person's celestial self and 13th helix is established and adequate.

Refer to Appendix II on how to test a number. The percentage will automatically be included in the reprogramming.

15. TEST the percentage of cohabitation of light and darkness.

16. TEST if there is a bridge between the darkness, the light and the 13th helix.

17. TEST if the reconnection could cause a disorder due to the electromagnetic fields of the 13th helix and if it must be reajusted to be tolerated.

The answer must be YES. If it isn't, this data will automatically be included in the reprogramming.

18. TEST if the 13th helix is at zero point.

Before installing the program, it may be necessary to enter other data.

19. TEST if it is necessary to enter other data in this program before installing it. If YES, go to Appendix III and follow the instructions to test which data must be entered in this reprogramming. Then, return to the protocol and proceed to the next stage.

2nd Stage – The instal-
lation takes into
account all the data
found in the first stage.

2nd Stage – INSTALLATION OF THE REPROGRAMMING

Insofar as the command
is spoken out loud, each
item is integrated in the
reprogramming. Please
use the tone of voice you
would use for a prayer
or hypnosis as the DNA
responds to language
spoken in this fashion.

1. **SAY: *I COMMAND* that the 13th helix be installed in the nucleus of the master cell of the pineal gland in all lives and all dimensions.**

2. **SAY: *I COMMAND* that, from the pineal gland, this program reach:**
   A. the endocrine glands;
   B. the brain, the nervous system and the peptides;
   C. the cells, the intra and extracellular fluids, the interstitial void, the atoms and the quantum elements (quarks, muons, strands,...);
   D. all of the helixes, chakras, etheric bodies, and the soul;

If Point E tests YES,
refer to Appendix III
and find the area.

   E. another location (see Appendix III).

3. **SAY: *I COMMAND* the RNA to support and reconnect itself to the 13th helix.**

The original DNA
plan is the underlying
pattern that precedes all
genetic mutation.

4. **SAY: *I COMMAND* that the 13th helix return to the order of the perfect original program.**

5. **SAY: *I COMMAND* the speed of the photons and the structure of the DNA spiral to adjust themselves.**

6. **SAY: *I COMMAND* that the connection within the corpus callosum of the brain be restored according to the original divine plan.**

The telomere is part of the very structure of the chromosome. It is a protein found at the ends of the chromoso-mal strands in DNA that protects these strands. In simpler terms, it is the end of each chromosome. The telomerase is an enzyme that acts as the "glue" of the telomere.

7. **SAY: I COMMAND the perfect integrity of the telomere and the telomerase.**

Refer to Appendix VII for a list of systems.

8. **SAY: I COMMAND that any residues from old programs be eliminated through the appropriate systems.**

9. **SAY: I COMMAND that helix 13 be perfectly sealed.**

Refer to Appendix I for the definition of Merkabah.

10. **SAY: I COMMAND that the Merkabah be perfectly sealed.**

11. **SAY: I COMMAND that no radiation affect the DNA or RNA.**

12. **SAY: I COMMAND that helix 13 be reconnected until further notice, in the brain stem, here and now.**

13. **SAY: I COMMAND that the reconnection of helix 13 be perfectly tolerated and integrated and that this occurs at zero point.**

ESSENTIAL POINT in reprogramming

14. **SAY: I COMMAND that the power, the harmony and the purity of the 13th helix be installed in the DNA and be perfectly activated.**

3rd Stage	**3rd Stage – CONCLUSION OF THE PROTOCOL**

The installation of other data may be required before concluding the protocol.

15. TEST if it is necessary to include other data in the reprogramming for it to be effective, tolerated or integrated. If YES, go to Appendix III and follow the instructions to test which data must be entered in this reprogramming. Then, return to the protocol and proceed to Step 16.

This closes the protocol.

16. SAY: *I COMMAND that this reprogramming be tolerated and integrated, according to the original divine plan, in the frequency of love, even if our helixes have been deactivated in the past.*

This seals the reprogramming.

17. SAY: *I COMMAND that this regeneration be complete and sealed, until further notice from ... (the person being reprogrammed).*

The effects of reconnecting the 13th helix can be surprising, especially for people who tend to "float" and who have trouble staying grounded in their physical bodies. I asked my students to share their comments about the results obtained from several protocols. Nicole F. sent the following information regarding the first two protocols.

Re-establishing the 13 helixes gave me the chance to connect to a physical and emotional well-being never experienced before. The quietness, peace and serenity that followed were the rewards of years of research and work on myself. With regard to the activation of each of the helixes (Protocol 3), it can be said that life chose to put me in situations which ensured that the assimilation would be successful. These where like a friendly nod from life, whereas before… well, everything was so dramatic!

Marie D's experience enabled her to get in touch with aspects of herself that she had no idea existed.

For me, reprogramming my DNA, and becoming aware of the endless possibilities that opened up before me, was an incredible discovery. Without knowing it, I already had a few helixes that had reconnected before I started this work. But when I started to reconnect the other helixes, I understood what had been going on inside of me during the last few years. Up to that point, and for several years prior, I had a reoccurring dream in which I lived in a big house that had rooms I could not enter. I was thus confined to just a few rooms, which were quite gloomy and very cluttered. Reconnecting my helixes left me feeling that I could find the keys to open the doors of those other rooms. It was like *discovering aspects of myself that I had never seen yet! Once the 13th helix was recon-nected, it became easier for me to reconcile with life and accept its limitations here on this planet. I finally was able to get back in touch with a dream from my youth, one that I had come to qualify as utopian: the possibility of "spiritualizing" matter and material-izing the spiritual on Earth. Somehow, it no longer seems utopian to me!*

PROTOCOL NO. 3

Reharmonizing/Activating the 13 Helixes

At this point in the book, it is easier for us to understand that there are several ways to reprogram our helixes. Whether we are aware of it or not, the reprogramming of our junk or random DNA has already begun. As we have seen, photon emissions (light) that come from sources beyond our planet have their own way of positively influencing our DNA and contributing to the reconnection of our helixes. Thanks to the protocols, we also understand that we can influence this process through the use of conscious commands. The formulation of intentions constitutes a series of commands, issued by our consciousness, which influence the arrangement of our helixes, hence our DNA.

Completing the work in the first two protocols will probably have sufficed in convincing you of the power you have over your DNA. The 13 helixes, including the 11 that were disconnected and scattered, are now reconnected. However, not all of them are activated and harmonized. Even the first two, the two physical helixes, need to be harmonized to be 100% activated, since 97% of their genes are considered to be "superfluous" and inactive DNA.

Part of this reharmonization/activation process will occur on its own, naturally, as underlined by Nicole F on the previous page. However, we can accelerate the process by using Protocol 3. The objective of this protocol is to bring each helix to a level of activation reaching 100%. This can only be done if each helix is reharmonized, i.e. if all its aspects or elements are reprogrammed adequately. Helixes cannot be functional or 100% activated if they are not reharmonized.

The reharmonization and activation of helixes includes a series of elements to verify for each helix. The elements listed in the following chart are, in fact, indicators of the current state of our helixes.

TABLE OF INDICATORS

	HELIXES	1	2	3	4	5	6
1	% of activation?						
2	Remodelling						
3	Miasmas						
4	Curses						
5	Emotions						
6	Mental beliefs						
7	Spiritual						
8	Implant						
9	Allergies						
10	Infections						
11	Free radicals						
12	% of undulatory frequency of the DNA						
13	Hormones: pineal, pituitary, thyroid, thymus, pancreas, adrenals, ovary/testicle, hypothalamus, thalamus.						
14	Circulation						
15	Structural						
16	Holographic insertion						
17	Hole						
18	Misalignment						
19	Distorsion						
20	Fragments						
21	Imprint						
22	Repair						
23	Mutation						
24	Polarity/Duality						
25	Structure of the DNA + reason						
26	Alliances/vows						
27	Vulnerability/without protection						
28	Original cause						
29	Memory of the initial program						
30	Rip						
31	Scars						
32	Coded to love at ____%?						
33	Interference						
34	Sealed at ____%?						
35	Health code (Protocol No. 5)						
36	Programmed for success at ____%?						
37	Youth/longevity (Protocol No. 7)						
38	Other protocol						

TABLE OF INDICATORS

	HELIXES	7	8	9	10	11	12	13
1	% of activation?							
2	Remodelling							
3	Miasmas							
4	Curses							
5	Emotions							
6	Mental beliefs							
7	Spiritual							
8	Implant							
9	Allergies							
10	Infections							
11	Free radicals							
12	% of undulatory frequency of the DNA							
13	Hormones: pineal, pituitary, thyroid, thymus, pancreas, adrenals, ovary/testicle, hypothalamus, thalamus.							
14	Circulation							
15	Structural							
16	Holographic insertion							
17	Hole							
18	Misalignment							
19	Distorsion							
20	Fragments							
21	Imprint							
22	Repair							
23	Mutation							
24	Polarity/Duality							
25	Structure of the DNA + reason							
26	Alliances/vows							
27	Vulnerability/without protection							
28	Original cause							
29	Memory of the initial program							
30	Rip							
31	Scars							
32	Coded to love at ____%?							
33	Interference							
34	Sealed at ____%?							
35	Health code (Protocol No. 5)							
36	Programmed for success at ____%?							
37	Youth/longevity (Protocol No. 7)							
38	Other protocol							

The following definitions provide more explanations for some indicators listed in the previous page.

DEFINITIONS OF ELEMENTS OR INDICATORS

Alliances/vows	Certain vows or spiritual alliances can sometimes prevent us from activating a helix and its level of consciousness.
Coded to love at ____ %	We have lost the ability to love fully in all the mutations of the DNA. However it can be reinstalled in this protocol. Test the percentage which has been lost.
Curses	In some cases, rage (or any other strong emotion) can be such that its emotional charge acts like a curse. Verify if a curse applies here and if it was given or received.
Distortion	The electromagnetic wave of the DNA spiral is affected.
Fragments	Please refer to Appendix 1 for the definition of a fragment. Test how many fragments have separated themselves from the person and if they need to be brought back in order to activate the helix.
Free radicals	Free radicals are toxins that can affect the blood-brain barrier. The blood-brain barrier is a sanguine filter which only allows tiny molecules such as glucose to pass through the brain. Once it is compromised, it can have an effect on the pineal and the pituitary glands. They are involved in the installation of the reprogramming of the DNA and we don't want free radicals to impede the activation of the helixes.
Holes	Holes can be found in bodies of energy and could become an obstacle when activating helixes.
Hologram	Please refer to Appendix 1 for the definition of a hologram.
Imprint	Imprints are found on everyone and in all bodies of energy. Imprints can be new, from past lives or from the ego. They can be positive or negative, but some are no longer useful. Most imprints that are issued from the past will slow down our current process of conscious change. Furthermore, they could have been inserted by negative entities.
Interference	There may be planetary or stellar interference, which could affect the activation.
Memory of original programming	We need to make sure at this point that we reinsert the perfect original program.
Miasmas	Please refer to Appendix 1 for the definition of a miasma.
Misalignment	The alignment of the frequency of consciousness is faulty and creates a resonance that prevents us from being in harmony and from having a sense of personal fulfilment.
Mutation	Genetic mutation can affect the helixes.
Original cause	The original cause is directly linked to the loss of the original divine program in our genetic code.
Remodelling	There is something in the DNA's original plan that has been changed and must be remodelled.
Structural	Certain physical problems can affect the activation of helixes. The word "structural" designates a condition which relates to the spine. For example, if someone is blocked in the back, this can affect or block vibratory energy.

Each element and definition in the chart is an indicator that allows you to check the state of functioning of each of the diagnosed helixes. A word of warning is needed here. **You must not attempt to include all the helixes, or all indicators for a given helix, in one single session because the nervous system cannot take it.** Harmonizing and activating of the helixes is a process that produces effects—you will notice this yourself—and requires that you proceed gradually to allow your body to adjust adequately. For this reason, you will need to do several sessions with Protocol 3.

The first few questions of the protocol will guide you in knowing which helix needs to be treated and how many indicators can be included in each session. Step 1 will help you determine which helix you will work on during the course of the session, i.e. which helix will be reprogrammed so that it is harmonized and its level of activation increased. Step 2 will help you test the current percentage of activation of the helix before completing the protocol.

Step 3 of Protocol 3 will accurately advise you on what you may include in the reprogramming process. In order to check Step 3A, simply refer to the List of Indicators and test each line (each indicator) by asking the following question: "Does this indicator need to be reharmonized?" Note each "Yes" since this will give you the big picture on the state of that particular helix. Step 3B will help you determine the number of indicators that can be treated during the session in progress, and finally, Step 3C will allow you to identify precisely which indicators will be included and in which order they will be handled.

At the end of the protocol, you can re-check the helix's percentage of activation, which may have changed. It may have increased or decreased. This does not mean that you have failed. On the contrary, it means that for the reharmonization to be tolerated, the level of activation of the helix may need to be temporarily lowered to give your body a chance to adjust. In my experience, by checking the activation of the helix several days or weeks later, you will notice that it has increased from what it had been before you began the process of reprogramming. It is also possible that increasing the level of activation may need to wait until after you have reharmonized and reactivated another helix since the body and all helixes form a whole.

Do not become discouraged by the number of elements on the list of indicators. Each helix has its own specificity and functions. Therefore, it is important to test each element for each helix. However, it is just as important to proceed slowly and have faith in your innate intelligence, which communicates with you via your testing method (kinesiology or otherwise). The test will tell you in which order you need to proceed so that activation is done adequately. Even if you only focus on one element for a given helix per session, you will quickly notice changes in yourself, whether physical, emotional, psychological or spiritual. And even if your basic intention for each session refers to a single element of a helix, your innate intelligence will understand that your ultimate intention is to fully harmonize and reactivate all your helixes, and it will adjust your programs accordingly.

Go ahead, have fun reharmonizing and reactivating all of your helixes!

PROTOCOL NO. 3

Reharmonizing / Activating the 13 Helixes

1ˢᵗ Stage of Protocol

Identifies the object of the protocol as well as the data to be included in the repromming process.

The percentage of activation is rarely 100%. As time goes on, the percentage may vary according to the work you have accomplished in the previous session.

Refer to the Table of Indicators on page 68 and test each element. IMPORTANT: do not treat more than three elements at a time during a reprogramming session.

1ˢᵗ Stage – PREPARATION

Before beginning to test, set your intent by saying: **I choose to be at zero point even if I don't know how.**

Use kinesiology (or another testing tool) to find the answers. Data thus obtained will be automatically processed by the body's innate intelligence and the genetic code's consciousness, in accordance with your intention.

1. **TEST which helix needs to be activated and reharmonized during this reprogramming.**

2. **TEST the percentage of activation of this helix.**

3. **A. TEST which element(s) of the Table of Indicators must be reharmonized on this helix.**
   B. TEST the number of elements that must be included in the present reprogramming.
   C. TEST which specific elements will be treated in this reprogramming and the order in which to treat them.
   IMPORTANT: If more than one element is treated, perform Steps 4 to 9 of the 1ˢᵗ Stage (Preparation) for each element separately, in the order indicated in No. 3C above. Once all the elements are treated, proceed to the 2ⁿᵈ Stage (Installation). *Example: At No. 3A, 6 elements were identified. No. 3B indicates that you can include two of these elements in this reprogramming. At No. 3C, test which ones among those found at No. 3A to include, then test in which order to treat them. Then, proceed with Nos. 4 to 9 for each of these elements, treating them in the order indicated.*

73

Refer to Appendix II on how to test a number.

4. **A. TEST how many items from Appendix III must be entered in the reprogramming for the chosen element.**

Each time data from Appendix III is tested, it will be included automatically in the reprogramming.

    B. TEST each section of Appendix III one by one until the item has been identified.

Finding the exact DNA address is the MAIN PIVOT of all reprogramming. In general, the program is in one gene of a single chromosome.

5. **TEST if this program must be coded in a specific chromosome or gene.**
   If YES,
       A. TEST which chromosome (1 to 46...) **and which gene** (1 to 5,000+).
       B. TEST how many codons (1 to 30,000+) **are in this program.**

The original DNA plan is the underlying diagram that precedes all genetic mutation. If this information still exists in a latent form, it will automatically be included in the reprogramming.

6. **TEST if this program already existed in the original divine plan of the person's DNA.**
   If YES,
       A. TEST if it can be reproduced here.
       B. TEST if a bridge must be installed.

A theme or another program may neutralize the installation of the new program.

7. **TEST if there is a harmful program or theme in resonance (echo) or duality (polarity) that could interfere with the new program.**

Memories linked to former programs are capable of interfering with the new program.

8. **TEST if there are memories attached or linked to former programs that could interfere with integrating this new program in the DNA.**
   If YES, how many memories are there?

9. **TEST if this helix is at zero point.**
   IMPORTANT: Return to Step 4 to reharmonize the other elements planned for this reprogramming BEFORE proceeding to the 2nd Stage (Installation).

2nd Stage – The instal-
lation takes into
account all the data
found in the first stage.

2nd Stage – INSTALLATION OF THE REPROGRAMMING

If several elements were
chosen at Step 3, com-
mand that all be
installed at the same
time. Insofar as the
command is spoken out
loud, each item is inte-
grated in the repro-
gramming. Please use
the tone of voice you
would use for a prayer
or hypnosis as the DNA
responds to language
spoken in this fashion.

If Point E tests YES ,
refer to Appendix III
and find the area.

1. **SAY: I COMMAND that the program(s) be installed in the nucleus of the master cell of the pineal gland in all lives and all dimensions.**

2. **SAY: I COMMAND that, from the pineal gland, the program(s) reach:**
   A. the endocrine glands;
   B. the brain, the nervous system and the peptides;
   C. the cells, the intra and extracellular fluids, the interstitial void, the atoms and the quantum elements (quarks, muons, strands,...);
   D. all of the helixes, chakras, etheric bodies, and the soul;
   E. another location (see Appendix III).

3. **SAY: I COMMAND the RNA to support and reconnect itself to the new program(s).**

The original DNA
plan is the underlying
pattern that precedes all
genetic mutation.

4. **SAY: I COMMAND the codons to return to the order of the perfect original program(s), even if there has been an inversion of codes.**

5. **SAY: I COMMAND the speed of the photons and the structure of the DNA spiral to adjust themselves.**

6. **SAY: I COMMAND that the connection within the corpus callosum of the brain be restored according to the original divine plan.**

The telomere is part of the very structure of the chromosome. It is a protein found at the ends of the chromosomal strands in DNA that protects these strands. In simpler terms, it is the end of each chromosome. The telomerase is an enzyme that acts as the "glue" of the telomere.

7. SAY: *I COMMAND* **the perfect integrity of the telomere and the telomerase.**

Refer it Appendix VII for a list of systems.

8. SAY: *I COMMAND* **that any residues from old programs be eliminated through the appropriate systems.**

9. SAY: *I COMMAND* **that the new program(s) be perfectly sealed.**

Refer to Appendix I for the definition of Merkabah.

10. SAY: *I COMMAND* **that the Merkabah be perfectly sealed.**

11. SAY: *I COMMAND* **that no radiation affect the DNA or RNA.**

12. SAY: *I COMMAND* **that this new program(s) be installed completely, and until further notice, in the brain stem, here and now.**

13. SAY: *I COMMAND* **that the reconnection of the new program(s) be perfectly tolerated and integrated and that this occurs at zero point.**

ESSENTIAL POINT in reprogramming

14. SAY: *I COMMAND* **that the power, the harmony and the purity of the new program(s) be installed in the DNA and be perfectly activated.**

3rd Stage	**3rd Stage – CONCLUSION OF THE PROTOCOL**

The installation of other data may be required before concluding the protocol.

15. TEST if it is necessary to include other data in the reprogramming for it to be effective, tolerated or integrated.
If YES, go to Appendix III and follow the instructions to test which data must be entered in this reprogramming. Then, return to the protocol and proceed to Step 16.

This closes the protocol.

16. SAY: *I COMMAND that this reprogramming be tolerated and integrated, according to the original divine plan, in the frequency of love, even if our helixes have been deactivated in the past.*

This seals the reprogramming.

17. SAY: *I COMMAND that this regeneration be complete and sealed, until further notice from ... (the person being reprogrammed).*

We must be sure that we've had enough time to fully integrate the data before repeating the process.

18. TEST how much time is needed (days, weeks, months) before proceeding to a new harmonization on this helix or on another.

Please note that, as you work through this process, your nervous system will grow stronger and gradually stabilize. It will also adjust to each element of reprogramming. As well, many of your brain cells that had been functioning latently will be reactivated.

This is why I strongly insist on the importance of proceeding gradually. Make sure that, throughout the whole procedure, each element of reprogramming is 100% tolerated. Make sure you remain in your comfort zone so that your body and emotions tolerate the changes that will occur. Use this protocol regularly, i.e. once a week or every two weeks, until you feel that each element of each helix is reharmonized, and that each helix is 100% activated. Once you have begun this work, you may then use other protocols without waiting for the procedure to be entirely in place.

From now on, each time you use one of the remaining protocols, you will need to determine three points of utmost importance, which can be summarized as: "Which gene of which chromosome in the junk or random DNA do I need to insert the new program into, and with how many codons?" This is what we refer to as the true PIVOT of all protocols and as the *sine qua non* condition to the successful completion of any reprogramming.

PROTOCOL NO. 4

Installing a New Program in a Faulty Gene

As I continued my research in reprogramming DNA, the popular idea that we create our own reality was always in the back of my mind, inspiring me to develop a variety of protocols. I was profoundly challenged by the fact that genetic programs fundamentally govern us, whether or not we are aware of it. The results that my students and I obtained using these protocols have convinced me that this type of work is indeed a powerful tool for redesigning our reality, no longer blindly, without understanding, but according to our most legitimate wishes. Often, we take on a passive position in the face of altering our reality because our by-default programs encourage us to be powerless. This is why it is important to know how to replace these types of faulty programs, and why I have created Protocol No. 4, which explains how to substitute by-default programs with more suitable ones.

Each and every one of us has the right to try to let go of a program that no longer suits us. Therefore, Protocol No. 4 first requires that the programmer (you) clearly determine the location of the faulty program and whether or not it should be dissolved or placed at zero point before beginning to install a new program. Moreover, and this is one of the most crucial conditions in this procedure, the programmer must clearly determine the intention of the reprogramming.

Take, for example, people who think they are a bit overweight despite having a healthy diet. It is possible that their DNA holds a faulty program that prevents the body from burning its fat. However, it is also possible that their weight problem is due to a hormonal imbalance. Or, the extra fat could be a form of emotional protection established by their body's innate intelligence because of some malfunction in a system which serves to remove toxins from the body. These examples not only show the difficulty of identifying the cause of a problem that we wish to solve, but also the ease with which the protocols help us to reprogram our DNA.

In fact, programmers who wish to address their weight issues do not have to determine the cause of their problem in advance since innate intelligence always aligns itself with the basic intention, which must be clearly defined. In this case, the basic intention would be "to replace the genetically-inscribed weight problem with the ability to be slim while staying healthy." That person can then begin reprogramming using Protocol No. 4. In this protocol, the person will start by determining precisely where the faulty program is located (whatever the program may be), in which gene of which chromosome, and whether they should be placing it at zero point or ridding themselves of it. Thanks to your basic intention, your innate intelligence already knows your objective, and will therefore indicate (through kinesiology or another testing tool) the address of the faulty program in question; whether it be the cause of a hormonal imbalance, the inability to eliminate fat, or the impossibility of eliminating toxins. The rest of the protocol will then supply all the necessary data to establish the new program, which will allow you "to be slim while staying healthy," and to ground it at another precise address (a gene of a chromosome) with the number of requested codons.

This is how we can reprogram all sorts of faulty programs, such as the tendency to be overly self-critical, an allergy that occurs each time there is conflict, or a sugar imbalance in the blood, as in cases of hypoglycaemia or diabetes. All these are examples of faulty programs that can be replaced by new ones. Reprogramming Protocol No. 4 will help you discover how to remove programs that you no longer want from your DNA and replace them with ones that are more appropriate.

PROTOCOL NO. 4

Installing a New Program in a Faulty Gene

1ˢᵗ Stage of Protocol

Identifies the object of the protocol as well as the data to be included in the reprogramming process.

In this protocol, before installing a new program, we either dissolve the faulty program or put it at zero point.

Examples of faulty programs: diabetes, Crohn's disease, etc. We command by saying out loud – "I command (subject of command)." Example: "I command that (faulty program) be at zero point ..."

1ˢᵗ Stage – PREPARATION

Before beginning to test, set your intent by saying: *I choose to be at zero point even if I don't know how.*

Use kinesiology (or another testing tool) to find the answers. Data thus obtained will be automatically processed by the body's innate intelligence and the genetic code's consciousness, in accordance with your intention.

1. **A. IDENTIFY the faulty program** (for example, that of diabetes).
   B. TEST in which chromosome (1 to 46…) **and which gene** (1 to 5,000+) **it is located.**
   C. TEST how many generations are involved in this program.
   D. COMMAND that this program be at zero point or be dissolved.

2. **TEST if the faulty program and its memories should be at zero point or dissolved:**
   A. in all lives, all dimensions;
   B. in all etheric bodies and chakras;
   C. in the 13 helixes and the soul.

3. **TEST if there are implants, karmic imprints, transgenerational memories or miasmas that should be put at zero point or dissolved.**

Example: If the objective is to replace the diabetes program by one which ensures the proper functioning of the pancreas, or by a belief in a healthy pancreas, the new program can be a new mental belief (see Appendix V), a healthy emotion (Appendix IV) or any other healthy physical program (Appendix III).

We may obtain a NO for several reasons. We don't need to know why. Simply respect this information and proceed later on.

Finding the exact DNA address is the MAIN PIVOT of all reprogramming. In general, the program is in one gene of a single chromosome.

The original DNA plan is the underlying diagram that precedes all genetic mutation. If this information still exists in a latent form, it will automatically be included in the reprogramming.

A theme or another program may neutralize the installation of the new program.

4. **TEST with which program you must replace the faulty gene:**
   A. **First identify the program with the person.**
   B. **TEST if this new program is the one that must be installed to obtain the desired result.**
   If YES, go to Step 5.
   If NO,
   > **TEST which new program must be installed to obtain the desired result** (whenever necessary, test in Appendices III, IV, V).

5. **TEST if it is appropriate to install this program in the person's DNA.**
   If NO,
   > A. **Do not perform this reprogramming.**
   > B. **TEST how much time is needed (days, weeks, months) before testing again.**
   If YES,
   > A. **in which chromosome** (1 to 46...) **and in which gene** (1 to 5,000+) **you must install this new program and**
   > B. **TEST how many codons** (1 to 30,000+) **it comprises.**

6. **TEST if this program already existed in the original divine plan of the person's DNA.**
   If YES,
   > A. **TEST if it can be reproduced here.**
   > B. **TEST if a bridge must be installed.**

7. **TEST if there is a harmful program or theme in resonance (echo) or duality (polarity) that could interfere with the new program.**

Memories linked to former programs are capable of interfering with the new program.

8. TEST if there are memories attached or linked to former programs that could interfere with integrating this new program in the DNA.
If YES, how many memories are there?

Before installing the program, it may be necessary to input other data.

9. TEST if it is necessary to enter other data in this program prior to its installation. If YES, go to Appendix III and follow the instructions to test which data must be entered in this reprogramming. Then, return to the protocol and proceed to the next stage.

2nd Stage – The installation takes into account all the data found in the first stage.

2nd Stage – INSTALLATION OF THE REPROGRAMMING

Insofar as the command is spoken out loud, each item is integrated in the reprogramming. Please use the tone of voice you would use for a prayer or hypnosis as the DNA responds to language spoken in this fashion.

1. SAY: I COMMAND that this new program be installed in the nucleus of the master cell of the pineal gland in all lives and all dimensions.

2. SAY: I COMMAND that, from the pineal gland, this program reach:
A. the endocrine glands;
B. the brain, the nervous system and the peptides;
C. the cells, the intra and extracellular fluids, the interstitial void, the atoms and the quantum elements (quarks, muons, strands,...);
D. all of the helixes, chakras, etheric bodies, and the soul;

If Point E tests YES, refer to Appendix III and find the area.

E. another location (see Appendix III).

3. SAY: I COMMAND the RNA to support and reconnect itself to this new program.

The original DNA plan is for the underlying pattern that precedes all genetic mutation.

4. SAY: I COMMAND the codons to return to the order of the perfect original program even if there has been an inversion of codes.

5. SAY: *I COMMAND the speed of the photons and the structure of the DNA spiral to adjust themselves.*

6. SAY: *I COMMAND that the connection within the corpus callosum of the brain be restored according to the original divine plan.*

The telomere is part of the very structure of the chromosome. It is a protein found at the ends of the chromosomal strands in DNA that protects these strands. In simpler terms, it is the end of each chromosome. The telomerase is an enzyme that acts as the "glue" of the telomere.

7. SAY: *I COMMAND the perfect integrity of the telomere and the telomerase.*

Refer to Appendix VII for a list of systems.

8. SAY: *I COMMAND that any residues from old programs be eliminated through the appropriate systems.*

9. SAY: *I COMMAND that this program be perfectly sealed.*

Refer to Appendix I for the definition of Merkabah.

10. SAY: *I COMMAND that the Merkabah be perfectly sealed.*

11. SAY: *I COMMAND that no radiation affect the DNA or RNA.*

12. SAY: *I COMMAND that this new program be installed completely, and until further notice, in the brain stem, here and now.*

13. SAY: *I COMMAND that the reconnection of this new program be perfectly tolerated and integrated and that this occurs at zero point.*

ESSENTIAL POINT in reprogramming

14. SAY: *I COMMAND that the power, the harmony and the purity of this new program be installed in the DNA and be perfectly activated.*

83

3rd Stage	**3rd Stage – CONCLUSION OF THE PROTOCOL**

The installation of other data may be required before concluding the protocol.

15. TEST if it is necessary to include other data in the reprogramming for it to be effective, tolerated or integrated. If YES, go to Appendix III and follow the instructions to test which data must be entered in this reprogramming. Then, return to the protocol and proceed to Step 16.

This closes the protocol.

16. SAY: *I COMMAND that this reprogramming be tolerated and integrated, according to the original divine plan, in the frequency of love, even if our helixes have been deactivated in the past.*

This seals the reprogramming.

17. SAY: *I COMMAND that this regeneration be complete and sealed, until further notice from ... (the person being reprogrammed).*

Hélène C. offered eloquent testimony about the use of Protocol No. 4. With her permission, I share it with you.

Up to now, I have used different techniques with my clients. However, the direct work on DNA using kinesiology has shown me that there are no limits and that results can be achieved quickly. You can see with your own eyes a physical transformation occurring, including a change in the client's energy level.

Working with people's DNA allows them to energetically reconnect with themselves. For a therapist, witnessing a client glow with contentment has to be the most precious gift. Each case is both different and extraordinary. For example, I saw a person with a high level of triglycerides and cholesterol regain adequate balance with the correction of a faulty gene using kinesiology. In a later medical examination, her cholesterol levels had become normal.

PROTOCOL NO. 5

Installing a New Health Code

In Chapter 1, I quickly mentioned that DNA's nucleic acids (A, T, G and C) combine in pairs and that those pairs re-combine in sets of three to form codons. For example, the set "AT CG GC" is a codon, and is one of 64 possible combinations. I also said that, out of those 64 possible combinations, only 20 are active in humans and that there are three more which we use as code releasers or switches. All the other codons have always been considered, by the scientific world, as being inactive and relics of our genetic past.

And yet, children are currently being born with 24 active combinations instead of 20. These children were born with AIDS but are now completely cured! The four additional new codons seem to form a program or code of perfect health. Moreover, since this four-codon program currently exists in the human gene pool, it thus becomes available to the rest of the human race. In other words, when I read this information about these thousands of children in the world, I understood that we could also install this new program in our DNA. I called it the "health code" and it is made up of only four codons. The following is the protocol that I developed to install the health code in our genes.

PROTOCOL NO. 5

Installing a New Health Code

1st Stage of Protocol

1st Stage – PREPARATION

Identifies the object of the protocol as well as the data to be included in the reprogramming process.

Before beginning to test, set your intent by saying: *I choose to be at zero point even if I don't know how.*

Use kinesiology (or another testing tool) to find the answers. Data thus obtained will be automatically processed by the body's innate intelligence and the genetic code's consciousness, in accordance with your intention.

1. **TEST if it is appropriate to install a program which provides access to perfect health**
   A. in general, OR
   B. in regard to a particular situation to be included in this session.
       If YES,
          TEST which specific situation.

Refer to Appendix II on how to test a number.

Finding the exact DNA address is the MAIN PIVOT of all reprogramming.

2. **A. TEST in which chromosome** (1 to 46…) **and in which gene** (1 to 5,000+) **the health code must be entered.**

The health code could include 4 codons, as is the case with the new children.

   B. TEST if the health code has 4 codons.
       If NO, TEST how many codons (1 to 30,000+) **it has.**

The combinations which do not work will be automatically enterd in the reprogramming.

3. **TEST if there is (are) one (or many) combination(s) that does (do) not work.**

Test each of the elements (A to K).

The data found here serves to build the new program.

4. **TEST if the person has the genetic code that allow him/her to:**
   A. **rest without being sick;**
   B. **change frequency without being sick;**
   C. **be loved without being sick;**
   D. **live with perfect health;**
   E. **be in his/her body without being sick;**
   F. **trust his/her body so that it can be healthy;**
   G. **stop and think without being sick;**
   H. **accept to be cared for without being sick;**
   I. **be tired without being sick;**
   J. **be part of his/her genetic family without being sick;**
   K. **any mental or emotional wound** (see Appendix IV or V) **without being sick.**

The original DNA plan is the underlying diagram that precedes all genetic mutation. If this information still exists in a latent form, it will automatically be included in the reprogramming.

5. **TEST if the health code already existed in the original divine plan of the person's DNA.**
   If YES,
   A. **TEST if it can be reproduced here.**
   B. **TEST if a bridge must be installed.**

A theme or another program may neutralize the installation of the new program.

6. **TEST if there is a harmful program or theme in resonance (echo) or duality (polarity) that could interfere with the new program.**

Memories of former programs are capable of interfering with the new program.

7. **TEST if there are memories attached or linked to the fear of getting sick again (or of a family member getting sick again) or to another pro-sickness program. If YES, how many memories are there?**

8. **TEST if there is a blockage that stops it from being 100% sealed.**

9. **TEST if the health code is active on the 13 helixes.**

The answer must be NO. If it isn't, this data will automatically be included in the reprogramming.

10. **TEST if there are miasmas that block the installation of one or many of the codons.**

11. **TEST the integrity of the RNA and of the immune response mechanism.**

Before installing the program, it may be necessary to input other data.

12. **TEST if it is necessary to enter other data in this program prior to its installation.** If YES, go to Appendix III and follow the instructions to test which data must be entered in this reprogramming. Then, return to the protocol and proceed to the next stage.

2nd Stage – The installation takes into account all the data found in the first stage.

2nd Stage – INSTALLATION OF THE REPROGRAMMING

Insofar as the command is spoken out loud, each item is integrated in the reprogramming. Please use the tone of voice you would use for prayer or hypnosis as DNA responds to language spoken in this fashion.

1. **SAY: *I COMMAND* that this new program be installed in the nucleus of the master cell of the pineal gland in all lives and all dimensions.**

2. **SAY: *I COMMAND* that, from the pineal gland, this program reach:**
   A. **the endocrine glands;**
   B. **the brain, the nervous system and the peptides;**
   C. **the cells, the intra and extracellular fluids, the interstitial void, the atoms and the quantum elements (quarks, muons, strands, etc.);**
   D. **all of the helixes, chakras and etheric bodies, and the soul;**

If Point E tests YES, refer to Appendix III and find the area.

   E. **another location** (see Appendix III).

3. **SAY: *I COMMAND* the RNA to support and reconnect itself to this new program.**

4. **SAY: *I COMMAND* the speed of the photons and the structure of the DNA spiral to adjust themselves.**

5. **SAY: *I COMMAND* that the connection within the corpus callosum of the brain be restored according to the original divine plan.**

The telomere is part of the very structure of the chromosome. It is a protein found at the ends of the chromosomal strands in DNA that protects these strands. In simpler terms, it is the end of each chromosome. The telomerase is an enzyme that acts as the "glue" of the telomere.

6. **SAY: *I COMMAND* the perfect integrity of the telomere and the telomerase.**

Refer to Appendix VII for a list of systems.

7. **SAY: *I COMMAND* that the residues from old programs be eliminated through the appropriate systems.**

8. **SAY: *I COMMAND* that the program be perfectly sealed.**

Refer to Appendix I for the definition of Merkabah.

9. **SAY: *I COMMAND* that the Merkabah be perfectly sealed.**

10. **SAY: *I COMMAND* that no radiation affect the DNA or RNA.**

11. **SAY: *I COMMAND* that this new program be installed completely, and until further notice, in the brain stem, here and now.**

12. **SAY: *I COMMAND* that the reconnection of this new program be perfectly tolerated and integrated and that this occurs at zero point.**

ESSENTIAL POINT in reprogramming

13. **SAY: *I COMMAND* that the power, harmony and purity of this new program be installed in the DNA and be perfectly activated.**

3rd Stage	**3rd Stage – CONCLUSION OF THE PROTOCOL**
The installation of other data may be required before concluding the protocol.	**14. TEST if it is necessary to include other data in the reprogramming for it to be effective, tolerated or integrated.** If YES, go to Appendix III and follow the instructions to test which data must be entered in this reprogramming. Then, return to the protocol and proceed to Step 15.
This closes the protocol.	**15. SAY: *I COMMAND that this reprogramming be tolerated and integrated according to the original divine plan, in the frequency of love, even if our helixes have been deactivated in the past.***
This seals the reprogramming.	**16. SAY: *I COMMAND that this regeneration be complete and sealed, until further notice from ... (name of the person being reprogrammed).***

With regard to this protocol, Chantal C. sent me a very eloquent testimony on the efficacy of this new health code.

Since I've installed the health code in my DNA, I no longer get the flu or colds. I used to get four or five a year that would last five to ten days. Since then, I've had one that lasted two days in the past two years. It's wonderful!

PROTOCOL NO. 6

General Protocol for Installing a New Program

Protocol No. 5, in addition to allowing us to install a new health codon, also teaches us that we can install new programs in our DNA—not only the health code—without necessarily replacing a faulty gene. This is why I have developed Protocol No. 6, which I have called "General Protocol for Installing a New Program."

You may use this protocol to install any new program that seems appropriate for you. Let us assume that you have decided to change your career and go back to university to get a degree in Psychology. You pass most of your courses except for Statistics. You were never interested in mathematics and have always done just enough to get by in this area because you considered it a waste of time. But this time you absolutely need to pass this course to obtain your degree, but you find learning this subject particularly difficult. You could choose to install a new program in your junk or random DNA that could help you understand mathematics.

In Protocol No. 6, it is even more important than before to accurately determine your basic intention. Let me use another example to illustrate what I mean. We all know that low-voltage frequency emissions occur in our environment, including satellite radiation, cellular frequencies, HAARP frequencies, just to name a few. Physically, we are generally not aware of these frequencies on a daily basis. But everything indicates that they do truly affect us. Since our goal is to become the masters of our DNA, and consequently, of our being and our reality, we could decide to install a program to protect our DNA from these undesirable and foreign frequencies. All we need to do is stabilize the electrical frequency of our own DNA at a high enough level for it to act, if you wish, like a lock, making it impossible for low-voltage frequencies to penetrate and alter our DNA.

To install this new program of cellular blockage, you first need to determine what level of frequency is required to stabilize your DNA. A frequency of 1.1 gigahertz ("GHz") is right for most people, but it is important that you determine precisely the frequency that best suits you. Therefore, before beginning to reprogram with this protocol, you first need to test whether the 1.1 GHz frequency is adequate in your case. If you receive a "NO" answer, ask whether the frequency that you need is higher or lower than 1.1 GHz and proceed, using kinesiology, to find the frequency that works for you. Once you have found it, formulate your basic intention. For example, "Install a cellular blockage against low-voltage frequencies in my DNA by stabilizing the electrical frequency of my DNA at 1.1 GHz." Then check whether this intention is the one that will allow you to get the results that you were hoping for. In fact, it may be that the intention "to install a cellular-blockage program against harmful frequencies" is enough and that you need not be concerned with the 1.1 GHz frequency to obtain the desired results. Whichever form it may take, it is this basic intention that will guide the innate intelligence throughout the reprogramming.

Protocol No. 6 allows you to install all kinds of new programs providing your basic intention is clear. While I was writing this book, America and Canada were very afraid of a bio-terrorist attack. One of my students suggested I install a code that would "transmute biological weapons" in our DNA! Once your basic intention is clearly defined, follow the instructions in Protocol No. 6 to install this new program in your DNA.

PROTOCOL NO. 6

General Protocol for Installing a New Program

1st Stage of Protocol

Identifies the object of the protocol as well as the data to be included in the reprogramming process.

1st Stage – PREPARATION

Before beginning to test, set your intent by saying: *I choose to be at zero point even if I don't know how.*

Use kinesiology (or another testing tool) to find the answers. Data thus obtained will be automatically processed by the body's innate intelligence and the genetic code's consciousness, in accordance with your intention.

Example: Cellular blockage program via the stabilization of the DNA's electrical frequency at 1.1 GHz.

1. **A. Identify the precise program that needs to be installed and SAY it out loud.**
   B. TEST if it is the right program to meet the person's objectives.
   If NO, find another formula and TEST anew, until a YES is attained.

We may obtain a NO for several reasons. We don't need to know why. Simply respect this information and proceed later on.

2. **TEST if it is appropriate to install this program in the person's DNA.**
   If NO,
   - **A. Do not perform this reprogramming.**
   - **B. TEST how much time is needed (days, weeks, months) before testing again.**
   If YES,

Refer to Appendix II on how to test a number. Finding the exact DNA address is the MAIN PIVOT of all reprogramming. In general, the program is in one gene of a single chromosome.

   - **A. TEST in which chromosome** (1 to 46...) **and in which gene** (1 to 5,000+) **the program must be installed.**
   - **B. TEST how many codons** (1 to 30,000+) **it comprises.**

The original DNA plan is the underlying diagram that precedes all genetic mutation. If this information still exists in a latent form, it will automatically be included in the reprogramming.

3. **TEST if the new program already existed in the original divine plan of the person's DNA.**
   If YES,
   - **A. TEST if it can be reproduced here.**
   - **B. TEST if a bridge must be installed.**

DNA Demystified

A theme or another program may neutralize the installation of the new program.

4. **TEST if there is a harmful program or theme in resonance (echo) or duality (polarity) that could interfere with the new program.**

Memories of former programs are capable of interfering with the new program.

5. **TEST if there are memories attached or linked to former programs that could interfere with integrating this new program in the DNA.**
If YES, how many memories are there?

Test each element. It we get a NO for "all etheric bodies", for example, we can test to see in which body we must install the program.

6. **TEST if the program must be installed in all etheric bodies, lives and dimensions, and the soul.**

7. **TEST if there are miasmas that block the installation of one or several codons.**

8. **TEST the integrity of the RNA and of the immune response mechanism.**

Before installing the program, it may be necessary to input other data.

9. **TEST if it is necessary to enter other data in this program before its installation.** If YES, go to Appendix III and follow the instructions to test which data must be entered in this reprogramming. Then, return to the protocol and proceed to the next stage.

2ⁿᵈ Stage – The installation takes into account all the data found in the first stage.

2ⁿᵈ Stage – INSTALLATION OF THE REPROGRAMMING

Insofar as the command is spoken out loud, each item is integrated in the reprogramming. Please use the tone of voice you would use for a prayer or hypnosis as the DNA responds to language spoken in this fashion.

1. **SAY: *I COMMAND that this new program be installed in the nucleus of the master cell of the pineal gland in all lives and all dimensions.***

94

2. *SAY: I COMMAND that, from the pineal gland, this program reach:*
   A. *the endocrine glands;*
   B. *the brain, the nervous system and the peptides;*
   C. *the cells, the intra and extracellular fluids, the interstitial void, the atoms and the quantum elements (quarks, muons, strands, ...);*
   D. *all of the helixes, chakras, etheric bodies, and the soul;*
   E. *another location* (see Appendix III).

If Point E tests YES , refer to Appendix III and find the area.

3. **SAY: I COMMAND the RNA to support, and reconnect itself, to this new program.**

The original DNA plan is the underlying pattern that precedes all genetic mutation.

4. **SAY: I COMMAND the codons to return to the order of the perfect original program even if there has been an inversion of codes.**

5. **SAY: I COMMAND the speed of the photons and the structure of the DNA spiral to adjust themselves.**

6. **SAY: I COMMAND that the connection within the corpus callosum of the brain be restored according to the original divine plan.**

The telomere is part of the very structure of the chromosome. It is a protein found at the ends of the chromosomal strands in DNA that protects these strands. In simpler terms, it is the end of each chromosome. The telomerase is an enzyme that acts as the "glue" of the telomere.

7. **SAY: I COMMAND the perfect integrity of the telomere and the telomerase.**

Refer to Appendix VII for a list of systems.

8. **SAY: I COMMAND that any residues from old programs be eliminated through the appropriate systems.**

9. **SAY: I COMMAND that this program be perfectly sealed.**

Refer to Appendix I for the definition of the Merkabah.

10. SAY: *I COMMAND* that the Merkabah be perfectly sealed.

11. SAY: *I COMMAND* that no radiation affect the DNA or RNA.

12. SAY: *I COMMAND* that this new program be installed completely, and until further notice, in the brain stem, here and now.

13. SAY: *I COMMAND* that the reconnection of this new program be perfectly tolerated and integrated and that this occurs at zero point.

ESSENTIAL POINT in reprogramming

14. SAY: *I COMMAND* that the power, the harmony and the purity of this new program be installed in the DNA and be perfectly activated.

3rd Stage

3rd Stage – CONCLUSION OF THE PROTOCOL

The installation of other data may be required before concluding the protocol.

15. TEST if it is necessary to include other data in the reprogramming for it to be effective, tolerated or integrated. If YES, go to Appendix III and follow the instructions to test which data must be entered in this reprogramming. Then, return to the protocol and proceed to Step 16.

This closes the protocol.

16. SAY: *I COMMAND* that this reprogramming be tolerated and integrated, according to the original divine plan, in the frequency of love, even if our helixes have been deactivated in the past.

This seals the reprogramming.

17. SAY: *I COMMAND* that this regeneration be complete and sealed, until further notice from ... (the person being reprogrammed).

PROTOCOL NO. 7

The DNA Fountain of Youth

The protocols discussed up to this point have probably made it clear to you that, once you have learned how to reprogram your DNA, a world of infinite possibilities opens up. Protocol No. 7 builds on the previous ones.

As soon as human beings acquire enough experience to truly become creative in their lives and significantly contribute to the collective wisdom of humanity, their bodies and minds often start to deteriorate. The phrase *"If youth only knew and if old age only could"* clearly expresses this. Is it not illogical that the more we become complete, wise and competent human beings, the less our bodies allow us to take action? That as we grow older and have more resources, our lives are ending?

Regardless, we all know of people who, at 75, 80, 90 or even 100 years old, appear to have the same amount of physical and mental vitality that they had during their youth. It seems that these people are born with a DNA that provides them with youth and longevity. Since I live in a body and increasingly love life, and myself, it is with this observation in mind that I had the idea of creating a protocol which enables us to install a youth and longevity program in our DNA.

You will probably notice in this protocol that I have included in its unfolding a whole section relating to the state of love. I have done this because the more we are able to believe and to stay in a state of love, the younger we remain. For it is the duality of conflicts, whether they are interior or exterior, which significantly drains and ages us.

By re-installing the youth and longevity program, we are re-educating our cells to live in a state of love. This is the image that we must adopt and maintain in our new biology. Our DNA holds the main schematic of our inherited traits including our life plan. However, it also holds the codes of the history of the universe, including all relevant information on the reality of love. We only need to awaken or re-activate this code, which will then be more easily preserved inside each of our cells.

Several of my students have told me that they feel and appear younger since installing Protocol 7. Diane B.'s testimony about this reflects typical comments that I have received regarding this protocol.

Since I've started using medical intuition, I began feeling young again. I thought that it was temporary, but when I took the course on DNA, it became even more evident. It's really fantastic! You have to see it to believe it—or live it.

PROTOCOL NO. 7

Installing the Youth and Longevity Program

1ˢᵗ Stage of Protocol

Identifies the object of the protocol as well as the data to be included in the reprogramming process.

1ˢᵗ Stage – PREPARATION

Before beginning to test, set your intent by saying: *I choose to be at zero point even if I don't know how.*

Use kinesiology (or another testing tool) to find the answers. Data thus obtained will be automatically processed by the body's innate intelligence and the genetic code's consciousness, in accordance with your intention.

Refer to Appendix II on how to test a number. We may obtain a NO for several reasons. We don't need to know why. Simply respect this information.

1. **TEST if it is appropriate to replace the program of aging and death with the new program of youth and longevity. If NO,**
   - A. **DO NOT proceed with the reprogramming now.**
   - B. **TEST how much time is needed (days, weeks, months) before testing again.**

   If YES,
   - A. **TEST in which chromosome** (1 to 46...) **and in which gene** (1 to 5,000+) **the program of aging and death is located.**
   - B. **TEST if it is necessary to put at zero point or to dissolve the death and aging program (memories included):**
     - **in all lives and all dimensions**
     - **in all of the etheric bodies and chakras**
     - **in the 13 helixes and the soul.**

Before installing the program of youth and longevity, dissolve or put at zero point the death and aging program.

Refer to Appendix II on how to test a number.

Finding the exact DNA address is the MAIN PIVOT of all reprogramming. In general, the program is in one gene of a single chromosome.

2. A. **TEST in which chromosome** (1 to 46...) **and which gene** (1 to 5,000+) **the new program should be installed.**
   B. **TEST how many codons** (1 to 30,000+) **it comprises.**
   C. **TEST if this reprogramming is:**
      a. **in general, OR**
      b. **in regard to a particular situation to be included in this session.**
      If YES,
      TEST which specific situation.

The original DNA plan is the underlying diagram that precedes all genetic mutation. If this information still exists in a latent form, it will automatically be included in the reprogramming.

3. **TEST if the youth and longevity program already existed in the original divine plan of the person's DNA. If YES,**
   - **A. TEST if it can be reproduced here.**
   - **B. TEST if a bridge must be installed.**

A theme or another program may neutralize the installation of the new program.

4. **TEST if there is a harmful program or theme in resonance (echo) or duality (polarity) that could interfere with the new program.**

Memories of former programs are capable of interfering with the new program.

5. **TEST if there are memories attached or linked to the aging and death program that could prevent the integration of the new youth and longevity program in the person's DNA.**

6. **TEST if there are implants, karmic imprints, transgenerational memories or miasmas to put at zero point or to dissolve.**

Refer to Appendix II on how to test a number.

7. **TEST how many patterns or events are associated with the aging and death program.**

Commands are spoken out loud.

8.
   - **A. SAY: *I COMMAND that the program of youth and longevity be installed in the state of love, at zero point, beyond duality.***
   - **B. SAY: *I COMMAND that the links that permit using the energy of the state of love at zero point rather than the body's vital energy for the resolution of conflicts be restored at the DNA level.***

The process of resolving conflicts and critical situations exhausts our vital energy. We therefore ask the body to draw from the state of love rather than from its vital energy to resolve these conflicts.

Refer to Appendix II on how to test a number.

9. TEST the percentage of the person's capacity to:

    A. use the state of love at zero point to install this program ____ %;

    B. maintain the state of love at zero point ____ %;

    C. believe in the state of love at zero point ____ %;

    D. install the state of love at zero point in all his/her genes ____ %;

    E. use the state of love at zero point to create what he/she desires in his/her life ____ %.

Before installing the program, it may be necessary to input other data.

10. TEST if it is necessary to enter other data in this program before its installation. If YES, go to Appendix III and follow the instructions to test which data must be entered in this reprogramming. Then, return to the protocol and proceed to the next stage.

2ⁿᵈ Stage – The installation takes into account all the data found in the first stage. Insofar as the command is spoken out loud, each item is integrated in the reprogramming. Please use the tone of voice you would use for a prayer or hypnosis as the DNA responds to language spoken in this fashion.

2ⁿᵈ Stage – INSTALLATION OF THE REPROGRAMMING

1. SAY: *I COMMAND that this new program be installed in the nucleus of the master cell of the pineal gland in all lives and all dimensions.*

2. SAY: *I COMMAND that, from the pineal gland, this program reach:*

    A. *the endocrine glands;*

    B. *the brain, the nervous system and the peptides;*

    C. *the cells, the intra and extracellular fluids, the interstitial void, the atoms and the quantum elements (quarks, muons, strands, ...);*

    D. *all of the helixes, chakras, etheric bodies, and the soul;*

    E. *another location* (see Appendix III).

If Point E tests YES, refer to Appendix III and find the area.

3. **SAY:** *I COMMAND the RNA to support and reconnect itself to this new program.*

The original DNA plan is the underlying pattern that precedes all genetic mutation.

4. **SAY:** *I COMMAND the codons to return to the order of the perfect original program even if there has been an inversion of codes.*

5. **SAY:** *I COMMAND the speed of the photons and the structure of the DNA spiral to adjust themselves.*

6. **SAY:** *I COMMAND that the connection within the corpus callosum of the brain be restored according to the original divine plan.*

The telomere is part of the very structure of the chromosome. It is a protein found at the ends of the chromosomal strands in DNA that protects these strands. In simpler terms, it is the end of each chromosome. The telomerase is an enzyme that acts as the "glue" of the telomere.

7. **SAY:** *I COMMAND the perfect integrity of the telomere and the telomerase.*

Refer to Appendix VII for a list of systems.

8. **SAY:** *I COMMAND that any residues from old programs be eliminated through the appropriate systems.*

9. **SAY:** *I COMMAND that this program be perfectly sealed.*

Refer to Appendix I for the definition of Merkabah.

10. **SAY:** *I COMMAND that the Merkabah be perfectly sealed.*

11. **SAY:** *I COMMAND that no radiation affect the DNA or RNA.*

12. **SAY:** *I COMMAND that this new program be installed completely, and until further notice, in the brain stem, here and now.*

101

13. SAY: *I COMMAND that the reconnection of this new program be perfectly tolerated and integrated and that this occurs at zero point.*

ESSENTIAL POINT in reprogramming

14. SAY: *I COMMAND that the power, the harmony and the purity of this new program be installed in the DNA and be perfectly activated.*

3rd Stage

3rd Stage – CONCLUSION OF THE PROTOCOL

The installation of other data may be required before concluding the protocol.

15. TEST if it is necessary to include other data in the reprogramming for it to be effective, tolerated or integrated. If YES, go to Appendix III and follow the instructions to test which data must be entered in this reprogramming. Then, return to the protocol and proceed to Step 16.

This closes the protocol.

16. SAY: *I COMMAND that this reprogramming be tolerated and integrated, according to the original divine plan, in the frequency of love, even if our helixes have been deactivated in the past.*

This seals the reprogramming.

17. SAY: *I COMMAND that this regeneration be complete and sealed, until further notice from ... (the person being reprogrammed).*

PROTOCOL NO. 8

Repairing a Gene in a Chromosome

In the so-called "civilized" world in which we live, it frequently occurs that we are in contact with substances that can damage our genes. Whether it be chemicals, viral weapons, viruses originating from experimental laboratories, genetic food manipulation or the consumption of transgenic foods, we have all suffered, or will suffer in the future, genetic alterations that are not always appropriate for our systems. For example, we know that certain flu viruses can lodge inside a chromosome and affect certain genes. An infection can act as a carrier, i.e. once the virus is dead, genetic material that is left behind infiltrates the cell, penetrates into the chromosome and installs new protein codes, which act as commands for the cells. Erroneous genetic information can also infiltrate our genes, consequently altering the mechanism of cellular reproduction. Finally, the very structure of our chromosomes can also be affected.

This type of phenomenon may explain why certain changes occur and why we tend to blame them on bad eating habits, a weak immune system or even simply getting older. Protocol 8 was developed to allow us to repair our genes and our chromosomes, if needed. If you test that your DNA has been altered in any way, do not hesitate to use this protocol. You no longer have any reason to live with altered DNA.

PROTOCOL NO. 8

Repairing a Gene in a Chromosome

1ˢᵗ Stage of Protocol

1ˢᵗ Stage – PREPARATION

Identifies the object of the protocol as well as the data to be included in the reprogramming process.

Before beginning to test, set your intent by saying: *I choose to be at zero point even if I don't know how.*

Use kinesiology (or another testing tool) to find the answers. Data thus obtained will be automatically processed by the body's innate intelligence and the genetic code's consciousness, in accordance with your intention.

A vector left by an infection may have recorded new commands in the DNA. It must be cancelled.

1. **TEST if an infection has left a vector altering or modifying the genetic code.**
    If NO, go immediately to Step 2.
    If YES,
    A. **TEST in which chromosome** (1 to 46...) **and in which gene**(1 to 5,000+), **and how many codons** (1 to 30,000+) **are involved.**
    B. **TEST if it is necessary to put this vector at zero point or dissolve it.**

Commands should be spoken out loud.

    C. **SAY: *I COMMAND that the new commands installed by this vector be cancelled and that the genetic code recover its prior original integrity.***

There may be more than 5,000 genes in a chromosome. If no gene needs to be repaired, it is because the repair concerns the structure of the chromosome.

2. **TEST if there is an alteration or a modification of the genetic code, or a loss of genetic material.**
    If NO, go immediately to Step 3.
    If YES,
    A. **TEST which chromosome** (1 to 46...) **and which gene(s)** (1 to 5,000+) **must be repaired.**
    B. **SAY: *I COMMAND the repair of chromosome ____ and of gene(s) ____ , ____ , ...***

Test each word.

3. **TEST if a nucleic acid of the DNA or RNA is at cause:**
   DNA: • Adenine • Thymine • Cytosine • Guanine
   RNA: • Adenine • Uracil • Cytosine • Guanine

This is like a ladder made with sugar and simple phosphate.

4. **TEST the integrity percentage of the DNA spiral components:**
   A. Deoxyribose (sugar)
   B. PO_4 (phosphate)

Refer to Appendix II on how to test a number.

5. **TEST the integrity percentage of the DNA spiral.**

Histone is a protein which intervenes in the transmission of the genetic message.

6. **TEST the integrity percentage of the histone.**

7. **TEST at what percentage the transmission of the genetic message is being done.**

The telomere is part of the very structure of the chromosome. It is a protein found at the ends of the chromosomal strands in DNA that protects these strands. In simpler terms, it is the end of each chromosome. The telomerase is an enzyme that acts as the "glue" of the telomere.

8. **TEST the integrity percentage of the telomere and the telomerase.**

The chromosome may have been affected in its natural form. It is necessary to TEST the status of each different part.

The nucleolus is a spherical body, very rich in RNA and located in the interior nucleus of the cell.

The Golgi apparatus is a cellular organite universally present around the nucleus.

The mitochondria is the "energy center" of the cell.

9. **A.TEST the condition of the chromosome:**
   a) **wounded**
   b) **mutated**
   c) **impaired:**
      i.   **in the cells**
      ii. **in the nucleus**
      iii. **in the nucleolus**
      iv. **in the Golgi apparatus**
      v.   **in the mitochondria**
   d) **altered structure**
   e) **loss of genetic material**
   f) **foreign genetic material**
   g) **miasmas**
   h) **other condition** (see Annex III).

   B. TEST if one of these conditions affects more than one chromosome.

Translocation is a transfer or exchange between two chromosomes, implying that part of one chromosome occupies a different position in the other. Crossing-over is similar to translocation, but it arises when a chromosome intersects another during cellular division. This movement provokes a transfer of one part of the chromosome and contributes to genetic variability.

10. **A. TEST if there is translocation or crossing-over:**
    a) **from one chromosome to another during the cellular division of a pair**
       If YES, TEST which pair(s) is (are) concerned: AT, TA, CG, GC.
    b) **from one codon to another**
       If YES,
       i. **TEST how many codons are involved.**
       ii. **TEST which pair(s) is (are) concerned on which triplet(s)** (1 to 300,000+)**: AT, TA, CG, GC.**
    c) **of a nucleic acid.**
       If YES, TEST which nucleic acids are involved: A, T, C, G.

    B. TEST if a bridge is needed for the nucleic acids to return to their original location.

A codon is a triple pair of nucleic acids. Ex.: CG TA CG.

   C. TEST if you need to reintegrate the original order in the cellular reproduction.

Before installing the program, it may be necessary to input other data.

11. TEST if it is necessary to enter other data in this program before its installation. If YES, go to Appendix III and follow the instructions to test which data must be entered in this reprogramming. Then, return to the protocol and proceed to the next stage.

2ⁿᵈ Stage – The installation takes into account all the data found in the first Stage. Insofar as the command is spoken out loud, each item is integrated in the reprogramming. Please use the tone of voice you would use for a prayer or hypnosis as the DNA responds to language spoken in this fashion.

2ⁿᵈ Stage – INSTALLATION OF THE REPROGRAMMING

1. SAY: *I COMMAND that this new program be installed in the nucleus of the master cell of the pineal gland in all lives and all dimensions.*

2. SAY: *I COMMAND that, from the pineal gland, this program reach:*
   A. *the endocrine glands;*
   B. *the brain, the nervous system and the peptides;*
   C. *the cells, the intra and extracellular fluids, the interstitial void, the atoms and the quantum elements (quarks, muons, strands, …);*
   D. *all of the helixes, chakras, etheric bodies, and the soul;*
   E. *another location* (see Appendix III).

If Point E tests YES , refer to Appendix III and find the area.

3. SAY: *I COMMAND the RNA to support and reconnect itself to this new program.*

The original DNA plan is the underlying pattern that precedes all genetic mutation.

4. SAY: *I COMMAND the codons to return to the order of the perfect original program even if there has been an inversion of codes.*

5. SAY: *I COMMAND the speed of the photons and the structure of the DNA spiral to adjust themselves.*

6. SAY: *I COMMAND that the connection within the corpus callosum of the brain be restored according to the original divine plan.*

The telomere is part of the very structure of the chromosome. It is a protein found at the ends of the chromosomal strands in DNA that protects these strands. In simpler terms, it is the end of each chromosome. The telomerase is an enzyme that acts as the "glue" of the telomere.

7. SAY: *I COMMAND* the perfect integrity of the telomere and the telomerase.

Refer to Appendix VII for a list of systems.

8. SAY: *I COMMAND* that any residues from old programs be eliminated through the appropriate systems.

9. SAY: *I COMMAND* that this program be perfectly sealed.

Refer to Appendix I for the definition of Merkabah.

10. SAY: *I COMMAND* that the Merkabah be perfectly sealed.

11. SAY: *I COMMAND* that no radiation affect the DNA or RNA.

12. SAY: *I COMMAND* that this new program be installed completely, and until further notice, in the brain stem, here and now.

13. SAY: *I COMMAND* that the reconnection of this new program be perfectly tolerated and integrated and that this occurs at zero point.

ESSENTIAL POINT in reprogramming

14. SAY: *I COMMAND* that the power, the harmony and the purity of this new program be installed in the DNA and be perfectly activated.

3rd Stage

3rd Stage – CONCLUSION OF THE PROTOCOL

The installation of other data may be required before concluding the protocol.

15. TEST if it is necessary to include other data in the reprogramming for it to be effective, tolerated or integrated.
If YES, go to Appendix III and follow the instructions to test which data must be entered in this reprogramming. Then, return to the protocol and proceed to Step 16.

This closes the protocol.

16. SAY: *I COMMAND that this reprogramming be tolerated and integrated, according to the original divine plan, in the frequency of love, even if our helixes have been deactivated in the past.*

This seals the reprogramming.

17. SAY: *I COMMAND that this regeneration be complete and sealed, until further notice from ... (the person being reprogrammed).*

PROTOCOL NO. 9

The Decoders

Following a meditation session during the full moon of February 2000, I became aware of the fact that there were people on this planet with a life plan similar to mine, but who were able to understand and share concepts that I had overlooked. I read their books and could not understand why, with all of my years of research, I had not been able to recognize these concepts myself as I read their work. The answer came to me during a full-moon meditation. They had more activated decoders of information in their DNA than I had. By using kinesiology, I was able to determine that, at the time, the capacity of the most highly evolved people to decode new information transmitted on a planetary level had reached 32%. Therefore, I established a protocol for my own DNA that would increase the decoding percentage to the highest level possible that would be tolerated by my nervous system. A kinesiology test showed me that I could reprogram my decoders to also function at 32% without any ill effects. I have done this while developing Protocol No. 9. Since then, the ease with which I have had access to new information has been astonishing. In the following months, I have also been able to once again increase this percentage.

My students in DNA reprogramming have also obtained impressive results. They noticed, since using the protocol to increase the functioning percentage of their decoders, that they could understand new, and sometimes highly complex, concepts much more quickly. When they were in some kind of learning process, for example, and were flooded with new concepts, they could register a larger amount of information at once. Several also noted that they were finally able to learn a second language. One of them, Yves P., noticed that this was a very useful tool to help him be more in tune with his intuition:

"Back then, I had started reading Gregg Braden's book Awakening to Zero Point. *Although subjects on our planet's magnetism and its frequencies were of great interest to me, and given the fact that my professional training made me more familiar with the author's language, I still had trouble integrating the information and remaining focused on the book. After having increased the functioning percentage of my decoders, I reopened the book with much enthusiasm and with a totally new understanding. While exchanging ideas with friends on the book's content, I realized that I had in fact gathered quite a bit of information. My friends, despite being more knowledgeable than me on the subject, had to admit that they had not grasped as much information as I had."*

As for Chantal C., she enthusiastically wrote the following:

With the decoders, my intuition has become very strong and I have attracted new clients without having to advertise!

You should begin by first determining the percentage level by which you can increase the functioning of your decoders, taking into account what your nervous system can tolerate. If you get "only" 20%, do not try to go any further at this time. It is not worth destabilizing your nervous system in an attempt to go too fast. Use that 20% as a basic intention and follow Protocol No. 9. You can always come back later and gradually increase the activity of your decoders.

PROTOCOL NO. 9

Increasing the Functioning Percentage of the Information Decoder

1ˢᵗ Stage of Protocol

1ˢᵗ Stage – PREPARATION

Identifies the object of the protocol as well as the data to be included in the reprogramming process.

Before beginning to test, set your intent by saying: *I choose to be at zero point even if I don't know how.*

Use kinesiology (or another testing tool) to find the answers. Data thus obtained will be automatically processed by the body's innate intelligence and the genetic code's consciousness, in accordance with your intention.

We may obtain a NO for several reasons. We don't need to know why. Simply respect this information.

1. **TEST if it is appropriate for the development of the person being treated to proceed with this reprogramming now.**
   If NO,
       A. **DO NOT proceed with the reprogramming now.**
       B. **TEST how much time is needed (days, weeks, months) before you can execute this reprogramming.**

The functioning percentage varies for each person.
Refer to Appendix II on how to test a number.

2. **TEST the current functioning percentage of the decoders.**
   A. **in general, OR**
   B. **in regard to a particular situation to be included in this session.**
       If YES,
           TEST which specific situation.

This notifies the innate intelligence that the intention of the reprogramming is to bring the decoders to this percentage.

3. **TEST the functioning percentage that can be attained and tolerated by the nervous system.**

Finding the exact DNA address is the MAIN PIVOT of all reprogramming. In general, the program is in one gene of a single chromosome.

4. **TEST in which chromosome (1 to 46...), in which gene (1 to 5,000+) and with how many codons (1 to 30,000+) you must install the new program to increase the level of activation of the decoders. This will install a new way of thinking and allow the person to tune into new frequencies and new information arriving on the planet.**

5. **SAY: *I COMMAND* *that this new program also be installed in the intelligent consciousness of the nucleic acids.***

The original DNA plan is the underlying diagram that precedes all genetic mutation. If this information still exists in a latent form, it will automatically be included in the repro-gramming.

6. **TEST if the program already once existed in the original divine plan of the person's DNA.**
   If YES,
       A. TEST if it can be reproduced here.
       B. TEST if a bridge must be installed.

A theme or another program may neutral-ize the installation of the new program.

7. **TEST if there is a harmful program or theme in resonance (echo) or duality (polarity) that could interfere with the new program.**

Memories of former programs are capable of interfering with the new program.

8. **TEST if there are memories attached or linked to former programs that could interfere with the integration of this new program into the DNA.**
   If YES, how many memories are there?

9. **TEST if the program is well inserted at the level of the nervous system and the peptides.**

10. **TEST**
       A. if the soul understands this reprogramming;
       B. if the program is tolerated at the spiritual level.

11. TEST if the person being treated
    A. knows he/she has decoders;
    B. knows that the information is available;
    C. understands the information he/she receives through his/her decoders.

12. TEST if the vibrational frequency of the person being treated must change.

13. TEST if there are antigens that compromise the activation of the decoders.

14. TEST if radiation, miasmas, transgenerational memories or implants should be put at zero point or dissolved.

15. TEST if the increase of the functionality percentage causes auto-immunity.

For Steps 16 to 19, the answer must be YES. If it isn't, this data will automatically be included in the reprogramming.

16. TEST if the frequency of the new decoders is perfectly installed.

17. TEST if the decoders are installed on the 13 helixes.

18. TEST if the installed decoders are 100% in the state of love.

19. TEST if the decoders are perfectly sealed.

Commands should be spoken out loud.

20. SAY: *I COMMAND that new neurological pathways be installed so that the person can use his/her decoders at full capacity and integrate the new creative solutions in his/her daily life at the rate of 100%.*

For Steps 21 and 22, the answer must be YES. If it isn't, this data will automatically be included in the reprogramming.

21. TEST if the person is fully able to make new connections with the information now perceived.

22. **TEST if the speed at which the person can find new and creative solutions through his/her new decoders is at its maximum level.**

Before installing the program, it may be necessary to input other data.

23. **TEST if it is necessary to enter other data in this program before its installation.** If YES, go to Appendix III and follow the instructions to test which data must be entered in this reprogramming. Then, return to the protocol and proceed to the next stage.

2nd Stage – The installation takes into account all the data found in the first Stage. Insofar as the command is spoken out loud, each item is integrated in the reprogramming. Please use the tone of voice you would use for a prayer or hypnosis as the DNA responds to language spoken in this fashion.

2nd Stage – INSTALLATION OF THE REPROGRAMMING

1. **SAY: *I COMMAND that this new program be installed in the nucleus of the master cell of the pineal gland in all lives and all dimensions.***

2. **SAY: *I COMMAND that, from the pineal gland, this program reach:***
   A. *the endocrine glands;*
   B. *the brain, the nervous system and the peptides;*
   C. *the cells, the intra and extracellular fluids, the interstitial void, the atoms and the quantum elements (quarks, muons, strands, …).;*
   D. *all of the helixes, chakras, etheric bodies, and the soul;*
   E. *another location* (see Appendix III).

If Point E tests YES , refer to Appendix III and find the area.

3. **SAY: *I COMMAND the RNA to support and reconnect itself to this new program.***

The original DNA plan is the underlying pattern that precedes all genetic mutation.

4. **SAY: *I COMMAND the codons to return to the order of the perfect original program even if there has been an inversion of codes.***

5. SAY: *I COMMAND the speed of the photons and the structure of the DNA spiral to adjust themselves.*

6. SAY: *I COMMAND that the connection within the corpus callosum of the brain be restored according to the original divine plan.*

The telomere is part of the very structure of the chromosome. It is a protein found at the ends of the chromosomal strands in DNA that protects these strands. In simpler terms, it is the end of each chromosome. The telomerase is an enzyme that acts as the "glue" of the telomere.

7. SAY: *I COMMAND the perfect integrity of the telomere and the telomerase.*

Refer to Appendix VII for a list of systems.

8. SAY: *I COMMAND that any residues from old programs be eliminated through the appropriate systems.*

9. SAY: *I COMMAND that this program be perfectly sealed.*

Refer to Appendix I for the definition of Merkabah.

10. SAY: *I COMMAND that the Merkabah be perfectly sealed.*

11. SAY: *I COMMAND that no radiation affect the DNA or RNA.*

12. SAY: *I COMMAND that this new program be installed completely, and until further notice, in the brain stem, here and now.*

13. SAY: *I COMMAND that the reconnection of this new program be perfectly tolerated and integrated and that this occurs at zero point.*

ESSENTIAL POINT in reprogramming

14. SAY: *I COMMAND that the power, the harmony and the purity of this new program be installed in the DNA and be perfectly activated.*

3ʳᵈ Stage	**3ʳᵈ Stage – CONCLUSION OF THE PROTOCOL**

The installation of other data may be required before concluding the protocol.

15. TEST if it is necessary to include other data in the reprogramming for it to be effective, tolerated or integrated. If YES, go to Appendix III and follow the instructions to test which data must be entered in this reprogramming. Then, return to the protocol and proceed to Step 16.

This closes the protocol.

16. SAY: *I COMMAND that this reprogramming be tolerated and integrated, according to the original divine plan, in the frequency of love, even if our helixes have been deactivated in the past.*

This seals the reprogramming.

17. SAY: *I COMMAND that this regeneration be complete and sealed, until further notice from ... (the person being reprogrammed).*

I want to close this chapter by insisting that you do **not push yourself over your level of tolerance.** When reprogramming DNA, eagerness and impatience can easily lead to sickness or depression, which can be very difficult to live with. When reprogramming DNA, the objective is not to create chaos, but to follow a perfect plan.

This is why I absolutely insist that you correctly follow the protocols. Even if you use a tool of intuitive nature (yin) to reprogram, allow yourself to follow the rational and precise order (yang) established in the protocols.

To offer secure reprogramming, I have developed, tested and fine-tuned these protocols with a team of expert and experienced therapists. Our experiments, including those of my students, have proven over and over again that reprogramming can provoke physical and emotional effects that, on the one hand, may feel good but on the other, may be uncomfortable. Consequently, **do not over-stimulate your systems and your body by reprogramming too much too soon.** Following the instructions can only help you to regain sovereignty over your DNA in a harmonious manner. Before you begin reprogramming a new protocol, make sure that you have assimilated the previous ones. If you find yourself in doubt, use kinesiology or the tool of your choice to determine if you are ready to move on to a new reprogramming process.

Chapter 4

BEYOND THE DUALITY OF TWO HELIXES

The current planetary agenda is to regain our sovereignty and be done with dual polarization. Dual polarization means that if I create something from light only, I inevitably generate a negative creative force elsewhere. We must stop favouring one polarity over the other and go beyond both the positive polarity (light) and the negative polarity (darkness). In the course of our evolution, we have now reached the point where we must integrate both polarities.

Effectively, we are in a state of constant struggle between light and darkness, good and bad, positive and negative. That is the dilemma of the human incarnation. The Chinese have a proverb: "What goes up must come down!" History is full of examples of that nature. We constantly go from one polarity to the other.

The only way to stop this incessant oscillation is to be on the frequency of love at zero point. Our society, however, is not based on love and it is difficult to trace a period in the history of humans during which love prevailed. We can observe long periods of conquest and ease, but politics, conflicts and all kinds of wars seem to have predominated over odes to love! I think, and this is just my opinion, that the "love program" is an important one among many others that have been de-activated in our DNA. This love frequency, or should I say, this state of love, has nothing to do with Valentine's Day chocolates (although I love receiving them), or with the love that I feel for my sister, for example. **The state of love is a space located beyond the positive or negative polarities**. In this space, good and evil, light and darkness, right and wrong and all other expressions of duality coexist at a balance point called zero point. Zero point is not a neutral state. It is not static. It is multi-dimensional, in continuous motion, and in the midst of perpetual change. Zero point is constantly in motion because the positive force of light and the negative force of darkness cohabit without cancelling each other out even if they exhibit opposite polarities.

The best way to envision zero point is to imagine a balloon full of water, floating in the middle of the ocean, spinning and rolling in all directions due to climatic changes and the motion of the waves. Zero point is located in the middle of this balloon. The core of this balloon is always balanced despite all outside turbulence.

Although I prefer the sphere-like image, it is also possible to imagine zero point as a fictitious point in the center of a straight line with a negative and positive polarity on either end. At zero point, the positive force is proven optimal because its potential is activated by the presence of the negative corresponding force, both charges being maintained in a perfect balance. With this said, it can be imagined that two opposing forces can coexist in the same space without ever having to join, just like the north and south ends of a magnet.

Dual Polarization and Zero Point

When we are not in the state of love at zero point, we are polarized (on the left or right, in good or bad, in light or darkness, etc.) However, what happens when we accomplish a task, a project or an activity and we are polarized? We simultaneously create the opposite. What we undertake while polarized can be successfully accomplished and seem to give us the desired results. Nevertheless, when we take a closer look, we see that our accomplishments took more time, more energy and more stress than necessary. It may also be possible that the final result, despite being acceptable, is personally inappropriate for us. But, more importantly, the accomplishment, which is polarized, and therefore subject to the law of action/reaction, will automatically create, energetically speaking, its own, opposite counterpart. These three examples illustrate the price you must pay when creating without being in the state of love and working out of zero point.

One of my clients once said, "Every time I call light upon me and I experience something extraordinary, it seems that everything which follows goes wrong!" I have had the same experience. Each time I had a truly extraordinary trip, I had a hard time coming home. Each time I had an extraordinary spiritual experience, I knew that I would have to integrate it afterwards through challenging "lessons" or detoxifying myself or doing something of that nature. In other words, it seems like "sunny days are always followed by rainy days". Another example of this phenomenon is the "yo-yo" effect that occurs when dieting. First there is the period of goodwill, when people deprive themselves in order to become thinner, feel good about themselves, or to clear their conscience. Then, several months later, in spite of all their efforts, they regain the lost weight One of my clients confided that, over her lifetime, she had lost 200 pounds only to gain back 300!

Zero point means knowing the limits we have as humans and welcoming them with love. When we join light and darkness, we can enjoy huge, extraordinary and powerful experiences that are both simultaneously comfortable and tolerable because this union is appropriate and it generates love. The students who have worked at attaining zero point have frequently referred to the experience as a state of ease and well-being that feels effortless.

The more we choose to be at zero point, the more likely we will vary the scope of our experiences and we will experience new emotional states. This way of thinking includes more freedom and a sense of love. The rainbow of experiences that colors our world at zero point is much more diversified than the black, white and gray that we have had access to up to now! Suddenly, we are accessing new data, having new experiences, and achieving greater things.

I have realized that the attitude which goes along with being at zero point continually opens up my world to new horizons. I feel freer now that I am less polarized. It seems that my responses, as well as my inner states, are beginning to vary increasingly. I even experience sudden and happy flashbacks, just like that, without any reason. It feels good to have such different experiences!

You have to understand that placing yourself at zero point does not mean "letting go of something". At zero point, we let go of nothing. On the contrary, we try to maintain two different polarities in the same space. Let us take for example a person who said: "I do not seem to fit into the project that we are doing at work. I will just have to leave my job." When we examine this situation at zero point, we realize that "leaving" because we feel that there is no space for us is adopting a polarized position. Thus, it is preferable to use an intention such as: "I *choose* to be completely myself while doing this project *even if* I feel rejected by the participants." By using this approach, we neither abandon the need to be ourselves, nor abandon the work.

Another common misconception regarding the state of love at zero point is the belief that it means not having any boundaries and serving everybody. A client once told me how important it was for her to devote herself to a cause and to be of service to humanity. However, she was frustrated about frequently being taken advantage of by those whom she was trying to help. I answered that that was the consequence of working out of zero point. It is important to be at zero point in each and every decision that we make. If being at zero point on a certain day means devoting yourself to others, then that is wonderful. However, the next day zero point could be completely different since it is a position that changes. Our daily goal and weekly intentions are to live at zero point and are not about whether we should help others or not.

Being active at zero point is very pleasant. There are no limits and we feel more comfortable than when we are in a polarized state. The question is: how do we reach or get closer to zero point? **By working with intention**. For example, when you wake up in the morning you can state the following intention: "Today I *choose* to be at zero point *even if* I don't know how." You could also practice putting all of your daily incidents at zero point. The mechanic at the service station annoys you? You can change frequency by saying to yourself: "I *choose* to be in another frequency *even if* the mechanic makes me feel inadequate." Or, you are waiting in line at the store and you start to get impatient? "I *choose* to place this experience at zero point *even if* the cashier's slowness irritates me."

By beginning with these small daily events, you will accumulate experiences at zero point. Once you have accumulated enough of them, you will discover a new way of life, and, rather than being governed by old programs, you will start to have experiences that are more original.

You will feel replenished when you give yourself the chance to feel annoyance and pleasure as separate but simultaneous experiences. You are simply allowing them to coexist at the same time in the same space just like two poles of a magnet that create a magnetic field. **This field, which is created by the two opposing, coexisting forces, is referred to as zero point**. Some people may have the impression that I have no problems. Heavens! What about the morning when my son was about to leave for school to take three final exams and he blamed me for an incident that happened the previous evening? I completely lost it and started to quarrel with him. My partner got involved in our conflict and, as if that was not enough, my three-year old spilled his glass of fruit juice! It was intense! Finally, we stopped everything and discussed what was really bothering us and eventually agreed that we were re-living ancestral family conflicts. Therefore, we collectively chose to install a new paradigm with regards to the incident even if we did not know how. This new paradigm consisted in positioning the conflict at zero point.

My son and I then decided to place our issue in a state of love at zero point and give each other another chance to see how we would react when, in the future, we were confronted with the same issue. I held him tight and told him that we were wonderful masters for one another. Smiling, he replied that we did not always do such a great job as masters, but nevertheless, he cheerfully left for school. Several months later, the conflict, which could have divided the family, blew over and we are currently at peace with the incident. I must say that we did have several good discussions before reaching that level of understanding, which included dialogue and reiteration of our intention to put the conflict at zero point even if we did not really know how! This enabled us to resolve the conflict with serenity and calm, without having to work out a compromise. Not a day goes by that I do not reaffirm the intention to be at zero point.

We must also place the results of our efforts at zero point. In the aforementioned personal example, deciding to place the conflict at zero point in the first place would not have necessarily meant that the conflict would have immediately resolved itself. This is what I mean by "placing something at zero point and waiting". As long as a creative solution to a problem that we have decided to place at zero point has not yet been found, we must maintain both forces together, in each other's presence, without letting go of either one. In other words, we must establish and maintain the intention at zero point even in the apparent absence of results.

Maintaining zero point is to live as if we already had all of our helixes 100% activated. And each time we take the risk of living as if we had all of our helixes, we create an environment that is more conducive to love.

PROTOCOL NO. 10

The New Paradigm:
State of Love at Zero Point and DNA

I do not think that it is possible to reprogram our DNA and obtain the desired results without working in a state of love. It is true though, that in certain laboratories, scientists practice cloning unethically and without concern for the long-term consequences upon future generations. Therefore, I cannot generalize and say that, without love, DNA is inaccessible. However, I am convinced that, in order to access the junk or random part of the DNA and reprogram it, we must first tune into this new frequency at zero point. To be able to change our frequency and establish a new way of vibrating, we will have to install a new way of thinking that is located in the state of love at zero point between light and darkness. In other words, for us to go any further in reprogramming our junk or random DNA, we must position ourselves at zero point and include both polarities simultaneously. Since the new programs have allowed us to reconnect our DNA and replace our by-default patterns, we can now emit more light (biophotons). If we radiate this new light while remaining polarized, we might disturb the people around us. This is another reason that makes me believe that the state of love is essential in order to do genetic reprogramming which is safe for us and others.

Throughout the history of humankind, we rarely see reference made to zero point. But history is beginning to change. Even spirituality is changing and becoming more circular or global. The frequency of love is the new form which corresponds to the evolving human beings who have reconnected and activated their 13 helixes. This new paradigm may be our last chance to change history. Furthermore, to make it easier to choose this new paradigm, I have decided to invent a protocol that could help me access original ideas. I wanted to find new venues to resolve conflicts that have continued to be repeated from generation to generation. It is so draining to always deal with the same old programs. Therefore, I have developed Protocol No. 10, which will help us choose the state of love at zero point and consequently, choose a new way of thinking about our lives and its challenges.

PROTOCOL NO. 10

Installing the New Paradigm to Choose to Be in the State of Love at Zero Point

1ˢᵗ Stage of Protocol

Identifies the object of the protocol as well as the data to be included in the reprogramming process.

1ˢᵗ Stage – PREPARATION

Before beginning to test, set your intent by saying: *I choose to be at zero point even if I don't know how.*

Use kinesiology (or another testing tool) to find the answers. Data thus obtained will be automatically processed by the body's innate intelligence and the genetic code's consciousness, in accordance with your intention.

We may obtain a NO for several reasons. We don't need to know why. Simply respect this information and proceed later on.

1. **TEST if you must install a program permitting continuous access to the new paradigm - to choose to be in the state of love at zero point regardless of the situation (conflict, difficulty, problem, etc.).**
   A. **in general, OR**
   B. **in regard to a particular situation to be included in this session.**

If NO,

Finding the exact DNA address is the MAIN PIVOT of all reprogramming. In general, the program is in one gene of a single chromosome.

   A. **DO NOT proceed with the reprogramming now.**
   B. **TEST how much time is needed (days, weeks, months) before you can test again.**

If YES,
   A. **TEST in which chromosome** (1 to 46…) **and in which gene** (1 to 5,000+) **you must install this new program and**
   B. **TEST how many codons** (1 to 30,000+) **it comprises.**

The original DNA plan is the underlying diagram that precedes all genetic mutation. If this information still exists in a latent form, it will automatically be included in the reprogramming.

2. **TEST if the new program once existed in the original divine plan of the person's DNA.**
   If YES,
   A. **TEST if it can be reproduced here.**
   B. **TEST if a bridge must be installed.**

A theme or another program may neutralize the installation of the new program.

3. TEST if there is a harmful program or theme in resonance (echo) or duality (polarity) that could interfere with the new program.

Memories of former programs are capable of interfering with the new program.

4. TEST if there are memories attached or linked to former programs that could prevent the integration of this new program in the DNA.
If YES, how many memories are there?

The answer must be YES. If it isn't, this data will automatically be included in the reprogramming.

5. A. TEST the percentage at which the new paradigm adjusts itself to human energy.
B. TEST if the nervous system tolerates and understands the energy underlying the new paradigm, or if it is exacerbated by it.
C. TEST if the new paradigm can be installed in the state of love.

These codons constitute a general program to let go of the old ways of thinking.

6. TEST if the program to release the former polarized thinking mode must be coded in a specific chromosome or gene.
If YES,
   A. TEST which chromosome (1 to 46…) **and which gene** (1 to 5,000+).
   B. TEST how many codons (1 to 30,000+) **it comprises.**

The answer must be YES. If it isn't, this data will automatically be included in the reprogramming.

7. TEST if the new codons are 100% functional.

Ask the person to say the sentence out loud and test while it is being said.
Refer to Appendix IV for a list of emotions and Appendix V for mental beliefs.

8. TEST if the person can say: *I choose that we make it this time even if I don't believe we can* **(or other emotion or mental conviction).**

9. **TEST if the cells have receptor sites for the new paradigm at zero point.**
   If YES,
   TEST if they are active.
      If YES, go to the next step.
      If NO, SAY: *I COMMAND that the receptor sites of the new paradigm at zero point be activated in the cells.*
   If NO,
      SAY: *I COMMAND that the receptor sites of the new paradigm at zero point be installed and activated in the cells.*

If we get a NO, this data will automatically be entered.

10. **TEST if the person being treated is saturated from the imbalance resulting from duality.**

While we once thought in paradisiacal terms, we now bear traces of losing this ability.

11. **TEST if it is necessary to put the emotional memory of the lost Eden at zero point or dissolve it to let go of a fictive perfect past and access the new paradigm.**

Commands should be spoken out loud.

12. **A. SAY:** *I COMMAND that a crystalline structure be installed in the left frontal lobe of the brain to anchor the new "state of love" paradigm.*
    B. SAY: *I COMMAND that both hemispheres of the brain balance themselves in accordance with this crystalline structure.*

The answer must be YES. If it isn't, this data will automatically be included in the reprogramming.

13. **TEST if the person can function in his/her professional and personal life even if he/she has changed his/her way of thinking.**

14. **TEST if the new paradigm is tolerated in daily life.**

Test each word.

15. **TEST if the new paradigm is well anchored in the physical and etheric bodies.**

16. **TEST if a new quantum particle for this new paradigm must be installed in the atom.**

Before installing the program, it may be necessary to input other data.

17. TEST if it is necessary to enter other data in this program before its installation. If YES, go to Appendix III and follow the instructions to test which data must be entered in this reprogramming. Then, return to the protocol and proceed to the next stage.

2nd Stage – The installation takes into account all the data found in the first stage.

2nd Stage – INSTALLATION OF THE REPROGRAMMING

Insofar as the command is spoken out loud, each item is integrated in the reprogramming. Please use the tone of voice you would use for a prayer or hypnosis as the DNA responds to language spoken in this fashion.

1. **SAY: *I COMMAND that this new program be installed in the nucleus of the master cell of the pineal gland in all lives and all dimensions.***

2. **SAY: *I COMMAND that, from the pineal gland, this program reach:***
   A. ***the endocrine glands;***
   B. ***the brain, the nervous system and the peptides;***
   C. ***the cells, the intra and extracellular fluids, the interstitial void, the atoms and the quantum elements (quarks, muons, strands, ...);***
   D. ***all of the helixes, chakras, etheric bodies, and the soul;***
   E. ***another location*** (see Appendix III).

If Point E tests YES , refer to Appendix III and find the area.

3. **SAY: *I COMMAND the RNA to support and reconnect itself to this new program.***

The original DNA plan is the underlying pattern that precedes all genetic mutation.

4. **SAY: *I COMMAND the codons to return to the order of the perfect original program even if there has been an inversion of codes.***

5. **SAY: *I COMMAND the speed of the photons and the structure of the DNA spiral to adjust themselves.***

6. **SAY: *I COMMAND that the connection within the corpus callosum of the brain be restored according to the original divine plan of the person's DNA.***

The telomere is part of the very structure of the chromosome. It is a protein found at the ends of the chromosomal strands in DNA that protects these strands. In simpler terms, it is the end of each chromosome. The telomerase is an enzyme that acts as the "glue" of the telomere.

7. SAY: *I COMMAND* **the perfect integrity of the telomere and the telomerase.**

Refer to Appendix VII for a list of systems.

8. SAY: *I COMMAND* **that any residues from old programs be eliminated through the appropriate systems.**

9. SAY: *I COMMAND* **that this program be perfectly sealed.**

Refer to Appendix I for the definition of Merkabah.

10. SAY: *I COMMAND* **that the Merkabah be perfectly sealed.**

11. SAY: *I COMMAND* **that no radiation affect the DNA or RNA.**

12. SAY: *I COMMAND* **that this new program be installed completely, and until further notice, in the brain stem, here and now.**

13. SAY: *I COMMAND* **that the reconnection of this new program be perfectly tolerated and integrated and that this occurs at zero point.**

ESSENTIAL POINT in reprogramming

14. SAY: *I COMMAND* **that the power, the harmony and the purity of this new program be installed in the DNA and be perfectly activated.**

3rd Stage	**3rd Stage – CONCLUSION OF THE PROTOCOL**
The installation of other data may be required before concluding the protocol.	**15. TEST if it is necessary to include other data in the reprogramming for it to be effective, tolerated or integrated.** If YES, go to Appendix III and follow the instructions to test which data must be entered in this reprogramming. Then, return to the protocol and proceed to Step 16.
This closes the protocol.	**16. SAY: *I COMMAND that this reprogramming be tolerated and integrated, according to the original divine plan, in the frequency of love, even if our helixes have been deactivated in the past.***
This seals the reprogramming.	**17. SAY: *I COMMAND that this regeneration be complete and sealed, until further notice from ... (the person being reprogrammed).***

According to Diane C., this protocol allowed her to miraculously recuperate from a serious accident.

In my opinion, the three-month DNA treatment that I received produced fascinating results. The psychologist who was treating me for a post-traumatic shock also noticed this. He concluded that extraordinary progress had been made during the four visits considering the trauma I had suffered.

To help us maintain this new paradigm at zero point, we need to remember the moments of darkness, depression or boredom that often follow the blissful moments. Choosing to place both darkness and ecstasy at zero point creates a new form of experience, a new feeling of control and a new kind of maturity which puts a halt to the never-ending wavering between polarities.

I suggest that you become passionate about this new way of thinking. I have seen so many conflicts that have been resolved using this new paradigm! Since I have made the effort to place everything at zero point, I no longer have the feeling that I am here simply to walk in the same shoes as my ancestors. I am less and less bored on Earth and find my daily experience increasingly satisfying.

PROTOCOL NO. 11

Integrating the Negative and Positive Polarities

In Chapter 2, I explained that, for our intentions to be magnetized and powerful, they should include both the negative and positive polarities. The way to proceed consists in creating intentions based on the model "*I choose...* (positive polarity) *even if...* (negative polarity)." The reason this works is that, when referring to energy, the positive takes all of its power from the existing negative parallel.

In order to really understand this mechanism, you need to think of a U-shaped magnet. The magnetic power of the right branch is directly proportional to the power of the left branch. The stronger the left branch, the stronger the right branch. In fact, a magnet with one branch stronger than the other simply cannot exist; it is physically impossible.

This same theory applies to our lives. The positive force is optimal when it finds itself in balance at zero point with an equivalent negative force. And from this balance at zero point comes the true power of creation. With a magnet which possesses powerful polarities, we can magnetize bigger charges. Consequently, when we decide to create in a state of love, it is best to do it with our two magnetic poles. For our purposes, our intention acts as the magnet and magnetizes a reality far better suited to our needs than the one we are currently in (our by-default programs). For example, in the intention: "*I choose* to have fun *even if* I am sad", "fun" becomes our positive polarity and "sad", the negative one. The essential condition is that there are two simultaneously opposed yet complimentary polarities. When this condition is respected, the simultaneous presence of both polarized charges creates a powerful magnetic field that attracts the desired reality. Events respond to the magnetic force of intention, and intention only works efficiently if it includes both polarities.

Before going any further, I must stress that the negative polarity of an intention does not mean that it is not "good". The concept of "negative polarity" is used in opposition to "positive polarity". The negatives and positives are conventionally defined as they would be in physics or in electronics. We speak of positive and negative poles of a current or of a battery. In this respect, the negative polarity "I do not have confidence in my body", in the zero-position sentence "*I choose* to be healthy *even if I don't* have confidence in my body", is not negative in itself for it could have been qualified as a positive magnetic polarity. The terms "positive" and "negative" are used conventionally to illustrate two different opposing forces such as the yin (traditionally negative) and the yang (traditionally positive).

Let us now consider that at zero point, beyond duality, a magnetic experience occurs in which positive and negative poles are simultaneously present. This leads us to say that in order to easily access zero point and go beyond the duality, we must have easy access to positive and negative polarities.

And this is what people who have been practicing martial arts for years can do. By integrating these polarities, masters of martial arts can accomplish extraordinary feats including defying gravity or healing with their hands.

Harvesting the Negative

Doesn't it seem that only initiates, wise people, gurus or enlightened masters hold the secrets of how to access cosmic consciousness? It appears as if they have discovered a power reserved only for the spiritual elite, and that normal people, such as you and I, are consequently left hoping that one day, with discipline, effort and whatever else, a miracle would allow us to also reach the same level of consciousness.

Then, in November 2000, while on a trip to California, I read an article about a Chi Gong master who had become known for healing with his hands. He had decided to share his secret through his teachings. He explained that, in the past, each time that a Chinese disciple attained the level of master, he shared only 90% of his knowledge with a chosen disciple before dying, bringing with him the remaining 10%. At the end of ten generations, a disciple had to follow all the evolutionary process once again.

This master also stated that at this point in time he had to transmit the totality of his knowledge to people in the East and West without any restrictions, since the human race was at a critical crossroad in terms of survival. The "secretive era" had come to an end. In his opinion, there are perhaps 20 people on Earth who are presently able to do hands-on healing using the same mastery he possesses.

In the article, he described the true essence of his secret. In martial arts, we generally think that the yin and yang energies (negative and positive polarities) must join like the black-and-white yin and yang logo we have all become familiar with. This, he believes, is an error since both polarities are not supposed to unite. They only need to coexist to stay in the presence of each other. He also stated that, in general, those who practice martial arts work solely with the yang energies, even if they think that they have united both.

When he grasped this knowledge, this Chi Gong master decided to try and integrate pure yin energy into his body. In its true nature, yin does not fuse with yang but rather pushes it away. When he tried to let the yin energy enter through his navel, without meshing it with the yang energy, the master simply fainted. The second time he tried, he fainted again. The third time, he managed to keep both opposed polarities together in his body. That experience gave him such magnetic power that, since then, he has been able to do hands-on healing. Furthermore, he no longer needed as many hours of sleep and he was in perfect health. By publicly revealing his secret, this master demonstrated his understanding of the next step of modern spirituality.

I knew, as I read the article, that life had just offered me a gift of great value. I meditated for long periods on this story and the new insight it brought to the energetic process. This secret, shared with such generosity and compassion, and that now floated freely into the collective consciousness, came to rest on fertile ground and the image that yin and yang had to coexist without neutralizing each other continued to grow inside of me.

Moreover, due to the reprogramming work that I had already accomplished on my DNA, an alchemical reaction occurred within me that awakened a dormant program. A revelation was disclosed. I understood that there was an available address in our junk or random DNA for the coexistence of yin and yang and that by simply reprogramming a gene in a chromosome we could allow the coexistence of these polar forces. I had just discovered a new route that did not require long years of discipline. I began working on a new protocol, which would allow us to incorporate the negative yin charge inside our bodies, and which would allow it to coexist with the positive yang charge.

The next step that I needed to take, in order to follow the example of the master, was to clearly define the yin principle independent of the yang principle. I needed to install a code so that my body could tolerate the opposing charges without me fainting!

I was very aware of the fact that, even with the best intentions, humanity would continue to live with sickness, negative emotions, etc. In general, most people believe that a conflict must amount to something difficult instead of believing that the outcome can be positive. Sickness, bankruptcy or conflict occur in our lives because we are unconsciously creating events that carry the negative polarity that we need in order to accomplish our projects. At this point in our history, the Earth is rich with all types of intense negative experiences. Everything that happens to us makes it seem as if we were incarnated on this planet to search for those negative polarities which allow our magnet to be at zero point.

However, negative events are so unpleasant, and negative emotions are so uncomfortable, that we constantly try to rid ourselves of them, either through therapy, compulsion, distraction, excessive exercise or any other behaviour that is prone to ease our stress. We then have to start all over again. Let us use a metaphor to understand the trap in which we find ourselves when we are out of zero point: The planet is a supermarket of emotions or of energies with a negative polarity. We enter this supermarket to "stock up on" negative charges in order to activate the power of our positive charges, but we immediately put the negative charges back on the shelf because even mere contact is too unpleasant. We arrive at the counter with an empty basket and must start all over again. In other words, we continuously create negative events in our lives because we need their negative charge to be able to activate our positive charge. However, once that happens, we do everything we possibly can to rid ourselves of the negative charge as quickly as possible. And we start all over again since we have not satisfied our need for negative charges.

Integrating the Negative

The only way to get out of this vicious circle is to accept negative charges, use them and integrate them so that they become one of the two charges of our magnet. It is difficult to maintain a very high positive charge on the magnet when the negative charge is so low. And, it is even more difficult to strongly manifest new realities if we do not have the magnetic force to allow them to stick to our life, like magnets on the refrigerator door.

As was mentioned previously, the Chi Gong master told us that the disciples of martial arts, who thought they had unified the yin and yang energies, were in fact using only the yang energy because these two energies repel each other and do not unite. This is exactly what happens when we refuse negative charges (yin).

However, this information gave me no indication on how to integrate yin. I discovered that later while I was treating a client. I was treating her for incest and as it so happened I myself had been up all night working on my own dysfunctional family history. Consequently, I had a lot of compassion for this client and her incessant battle with shame. I understood that with a past like hers, she would never be able to rid herself of the shame. At that moment, it was revealed to me that this shame, apparently never ending, was an emotion of extraordinary negative magnetic amplitude. I understood that if I could give this shame a DNA address, this client could then easily use this negative charge in her every day life. She would no longer have to remind herself of the humiliating events in order to use their negative charge to manifest whatever positive energies she wanted to magnetize in her life.

That morning, I understood, thanks to my courageous client, that I could help her to integrate her shame into her supermarket cart, or into her DNA. She would thus be able to take advantage of this process to increase her magnetic energy rather than feel constantly drained. Through this treatment, I started to develop the structure of a new protocol on the integration of negative charges.

As I reflected upon the nature of junk or random DNA, I realized that there were many such available addresses inside of us. We could integrate our daily negative charges and have immediate access to them without triggering unpleasant events. I have since reprogrammed many clients who have experienced an increasingly fast evolution.

Integrating the charges of our negative polarity experiences enables us to finally leave the supermarket with our hands full and access the power mentioned by the Chi Gong master.

The emotional stress and events that have marked our lives leave scars in certain areas of our bodies: the brain, posture, organs, endocrine glands, etc. It is as if those areas were circled with yellow tape, just like the tape that encircles the site of a crime. These are the "at-risk" zones to which we do not always have access. After incorporating the negative charge of these emotions with Protocol. 11, I noticed a vibratory regeneration occurring in these conflicting zones. Because of this, during each of my treatments, I now check to see whether these conflict zones can be reharmonized by the new negative charge.

I use Protocol 11 as soon as I need to integrate a negative emotion and I must say that, as I reprogram these new codes, I have been experiencing emotions I never felt before. I remember the first time I integrated the negative charge of "competition" towards a friend into my genetic code. This friend and I ended up having a very open and harmonious reunion. In the past, there had always been a subtle spiritual competition between us that made her censor her ideas. Because I am very sensitive on a psychic level, I was always aware of this and, when she left, I was often sad to have participated in this censorship and disappointed with my behaviour. On her next visit, I had integrated the competitive feeling before her arrival to see whether it would change things. The result was astounding. Our friendship blossomed and took on a whole new direction. We are finally beginning to write a new story.

Another example that comes to my mind relates to one of my clients, a businessman. He had started a business which made him the envy of many. With his people skills and his determination, his business reached the million-dollar mark. This man, however, had denied all the intrinsic negative charge of his success and each time he encountered a problem, he would explode with anger, screaming, and criticism, then go on to something else without being concerned by the negative emotions he had created through that behaviour. The manner with which he denied his negative emotions was linked to a by-default program that he inherited from his father, an extremely authoritarian man. My client made enemies who drove him to bankruptcy. Now, in order to achieve success in business, he has chosen to integrate the powerful negative charge of the "victim" emotion (awakened by his bankruptcy) into his genetic code.

Integrating negative charges is a powerful process. Imagine the intensity of the emotional charge of years of accumulated anger towards an abusive parent. If we could measure the energy volume of this anger, we would find an amazing magnetic force. Once this charge is integrated into the DNA, it becomes a wonderful negative pole that can be balanced by an equivalent positive pole minus the anger. From now on, our power of manifestation will result from using the dynamic between these positive/negative type of situation.

The magnetic charge of an emotion that, in the past, troubled and paralysed us, now becomes a force from which we will create what we want at zero point. We will no longer see the negative charge as something that we need to fight but rather as a force which we will use to create what we want in our life. This is why we will replace the "*I choose... even if...*" by "*I choose...with...*" From now on, this will allow us to feel that a new energy circulates and literally vibrates inside of us. We will feel how conflicts will rapidly be resolved because we will use them instead of fighting against them.

However, when we think of magnetic energy, Chi or vital force, we have to think of electricity, magnetic poles, the speed of photons, currents and ebb and flow of energy. One of the basic points of the Chi Gong master's message was related to the predominance of the yang energy. If you remember, the first time that this master allowed the yin energy to enter his body, he fainted.

Since the yang force has been predominant for a long time, one could therefore go into shock following the reprogramming of the protocol. To facilitate the realignment of both polarities and the change in intensity sustained by the positive force, I had to add an item in the program to the protocol in order to allow the yang to re-polarize itself (I must state that, before adding this element to the protocol, I almost fainted myself while I was doing it). To get through it, I reactivated in the junk or random DNA a lost program which allows the integration of both forces to happen at zero point. My goal was, of course, to make sure that the integration of the yin's negative force into the DNA did not destabilize the yang's positive force.

Before using this protocol, I had already accomplished many stages in the reconnection of my helixes and in the reprogramming of my genetic code. Therefore, I suggest that you first complete the protocols of the third chapter before undertaking the more advanced reprogramming of Protocols 11 and 12.

PROTOCOL NO. 11

Integrating the Negative Polarity

Important:

1. The people who are reprogramming (the programmers) must have experienced the previous protocols on themselves before undertaking this more advanced protocol.

2. It is important to identify, as correctly and precisely as possible, the specific emotion which the negative charge will integrate when implementing this new program.

1ˢᵗ Stage of Protocol

Identifies the object of the protocol as well as the data to be included in the reprogramming process.

This test is important.

The "precise" emotion is the one to integrate as the negative magnetic charge in the DNA in order to reach the objective. For example: a person who wishes to put an end to financial problems could believe that the negative emotional charge to integrate is "poverty" while the emotion here, would be "humiliation" or "weakness," etc.

1ˢᵗ Stage – PREPARATION

Before beginning to test, set your intent by saying: **I choose to be at zero point even if I don't know how.**

Use kinesiology (or another testing tool) to find the answers. Data thus obtained will be automatically processed by the body's innate intelligence and the genetic code's consciousness, in accordance with your intention.

1. **TEST if the reprogrammer (not the person receiving the treatment) can use this protocol.**
   If YES, go immediately to Step 2.
   If NO,
       A. Do not proceed with this reprogramming.
       B. Return to the preceding chapter and perform that (those) reprogramming(s) first.

2. **A. Identify the negative emotion to be integrated into the DNA by this reprogramming.**
   B. TEST if it is the right one.
       If NO, go to Annex IV, find another emotion and TEST if it is the right one before proceeding to Step 3.

We may obtain a NO for several reasons. We don't need to know why. Simply respect this information and proceed later on.

3. **TEST if it is appropriate to install the negative magnetic charge program related to this emotion in the DNA.**
   If NO,
      A. **Do not proceed with this reprogramming.**
      B. **TEST how much time is needed (days, weeks, months) before testing again.**
   If YES,

Finding the exact DNA address is the MAIN PIVOT of all reprogramming. In general, the program is in one gene of a single chromosome.

      A. **TEST in which chromosome** (1 to 46…) **and in which gene** (1 to 5,000+) **you must install this new program and**
      B. **TEST how many codons** (1 to 30,000+) **it comprises.**

The original DNA plan is the underlying diagram that precedes all genetic mutation. If this information still exists in a latent form, it will automatically be included in the reprogramming.

4. **TEST if this program already existed in the original divine plan of the person's DNA.**
   If YES,
      A. **TEST if it can be reproduced here.**
      B. **TEST if a bridge must be installed.**

A theme or another program may neutralize the installation of the new program.

5. **TEST if there is a harmful program or theme in resonance (echo) or duality (polarity) that could interfere with the new program.**

Memories of former programs are capable of interfering with the new program.

6. **TEST if there are memories attached or linked to former programs that could interfere with integrating this new program in the DNA.**
   If YES, how many are there?

The answer must be YES. If it isn't, this data will be automatically included in the reprogramming.

7. **TEST if the person can live outside the event that triggers this emotion and which provides the negative charge.**

The answer must be NO.

8. **TEST if the person still needs that type of event to have access to the negative charge.**

We must obtain a YES. If the opposite occurs, integrate the information in the reprogramming through intention.

9. TEST if the person can live outside of duality and integrate the two opposing forces without needing the triggering event.

For Steps 10 to 12, test each word to determine if they must be placed at zero point or dissolved.

10. TEST if the memory of this type of event must be placed at zero point or dissolved in all incarnations - past, present or future - and in all dimensions.

11. TEST if the stress related to this type of event must be placed at zero point or dissolved.

12. TEST if the miasmas that have entered or been activated by this type of event must be placed at zero point or cancelled.

Refer to Appendix II on how to test a number.

There could be hundreds, maybe thousands, of fragments.

13. A. TEST how many fragments have separated themselves from the person because of this type of event OR what percentage of the person is fragmented and separated because of this type of event.

B. TEST if it is appropriate to bring these fragments into the present at zero point and to anchor them in the DNA.

14. TEST if there is a familial pattern related to this negative emotion.
If YES,
A. TEST how many generations it goes back.
B. TEST if it must be incorporated into the DNA as a negative magnetic charge.

If Point F tests YES, go to Appendix III and find the place.

15. TEST if the negative magnetic polarity must be installed in the following zones of conflict so that they can be at zero point:
A. the brain;
B. the endocrine glands;
C. the nervous system and the peptides;
D. the cells, the intra and extracellular fluids, the interstitial void, the atoms and the quantum elements (quarks, muons, strands, ...);

E. **the 13 helixes, chakras, etheric bodies, and the soul;**

F. **another location** (see Annex III).

For Nos. 16, 17 and 18, the answer must be YES. If it isn't, this data will automatically be included in the reprogramming.
If you get a NO, go to Appendix V to identify the positive emotion.

16. **TEST if the person has access to the negative charge installed by this reprogramming.**

17. **TEST if the person can say YES to the corresponding positive charge. Is it important to know which one?**

This program exists in the DNA but it was lost.

18. **TEST if the person's genetic code contains the program to maintain the positive polarity in the presence of the negative polarity without neutralizing each other.**

The answer must be NO. If it isn't, this data will automatically be included in the reprogramming.

19. **TEST if the integration of the negative force creates a destabilization of the positive force.**

20. **TEST if the negative or positive force will undergo an electric or magnetic shock in this process.**
    If YES,
    > **TEST if it is necessary to install a code in the new program so that it can repolarize itself at zero point.**
    > **COMMAND its installation in chromosome __ (1 to 46…) and in gene __ (1 to 5000+), with __ codons (1 to 30,000+).**

Just as nothing is lost and nothing is created, the negative charges that we refuse can be used by other entities. Test if they must be placed at zero point or dissolved.

21. **TEST if the person was giving away the negative magnetic charge generated by this emotion to another entity.**
    If YES,
    A. **TEST which percentage of this energy was thus given.**
    B. **TEST if there was an alliance on this subject with this entity. If YES, put it at zero point or dissolve it.**

139

The answer must be YES. If it isn't, this data will automatically be included in the reprogramming.

22. TEST if the person can effectively manifest events at 100% without needing a difficult emotion to generate the necessary negative magnetic polarity.

The answer must be YES. If it isn't, this data will automatically be included in the reprogramming.

23. TEST if the person can integrate the new negative charge into his/her daily life.

We may have resolved an emotional issue and integrated it into the genetic code without the body knowing it.

24. TEST if it is necessary to install a bridge between the physical body and the negative magnetic charge.

25. TEST if the integration of the negative force is at zero point.

Before installing the program, it may be necessary to input other data.

26. TEST if it is necessary to enter other data in this program before its installation. If YES, go to Appendix III and follow the instructions to test which data must be entered in this reprogramming. Then, return to the protocol and proceed to the next stage.

2ⁿᵈ Stage – The installation takes into account all the data found in the first stage.

2ⁿᵈ Stage – INSTALLATION OF THE REPROGRAMMING

1. SAY: *I COMMAND that this new program be installed in the nucleus of the master cell of the pineal gland in all lives and all dimensions.*

Insofar as the command is spoken out loud, each item is integrated in the reprogramming. Please use the tone of voice you would use for a prayer or hypnosis as the DNA responds to language spoken in this fashion. If Point E tests YES, refer to Appendix III and find the area.

2. SAY: *I COMMAND that, from the pineal gland, this program reach:*
   A. *the endocrine glands;*
   B. *the brain, the nervous system and the peptides;*
   C. *the cells, the intra and extracellular fluids, the interstitial void, the atoms and the quantum elements (quarks, muons, strands, ...);*
   D. *all of the helixes, chakras, etheric bodies, and the soul;*
   E. *another location* (see Appendix III).

3. SAY: *I COMMAND the RNA to support and reconnect itself to this new program.*

The original DNA plan is the underlying pattern that precedes all genetic mutation.

4. SAY: *I COMMAND the codons to return to the order of the perfect original program even if there has been an inversion of codes.*

5. SAY: *I COMMAND the speed of the photons and the structure of the DNA spiral to adjust themselves.*

6. SAY: *I COMMAND that the connection within the corpus callosum of the brain be restored according to the original divine plan.*

The telomere is part of the very structure of the chromosome. It is a protein found at the ends of the chromosomal strands in DNA that protects these strands. In simpler terms, it is the end of each chromosome. The telomerase is an enzyme that acts as the "glue" of the telomere.

7. SAY: *I COMMAND the perfect integrity of the telomere and the telomerase.*

Refer to Appendix VII for a list of systems.

8. SAY: *I COMMAND that any residues from old programs be eliminated through the appropriate systems.*

9. **SAY: *I COMMAND* that this program be perfectly sealed.**

Refer to Appendix I for the definition of Merkabah.

10. **SAY: *I COMMAND* that the Merkabah be perfectly sealed.**

11. **SAY: *I COMMAND* that no radiation affect the DNA or RNA.**

12. **SAY: *I COMMAND* that this new program be installed completely, and until further notice, in the brain stem, here and now.**

13. **SAY: *I COMMAND* that the reconnection of this new program be perfectly tolerated and integrated and that this occurs at zero point.**

ESSENTIAL POINT in reprogramming

14. **SAY: *I COMMAND* that the power, the harmony and the purity of this new program be installed in the DNA and be perfectly activated.**

3rd Stage

3rd Stage – CONCLUSION OF THE PROTOCOL

The installation of other data may be required before concluding the protocol.

15. **TEST if it is necessary to include other data in the reprogramming for it to be effective, tolerated or integrated.** If YES, go to Appendix III and follow the instructions to test which data must be entered in this reprogramming. Then, return to the protocol and proceed to Step 16.

This closes the protocol.

16. **SAY: *I COMMAND* that this reprogramming be tolerated and integrated, according to the original divine plan, in the frequency of love, even if our helixes have been deactivated in the past.**

This seals the reprogramming.

17. **SAY: *I COMMAND* that this regeneration be complete and sealed, until further notice from ... (the person being reprogrammed).**

DETAILED EXAMPLE OF PROTOCOL NO. 11

Merely reading this protocol is enough to awaken important new programs that will integrate our negative emotions and allow us to increase our power within ourselves and in our lives. Since this is a more advanced reprogramming of our genetic code, I thought it would be useful to give a step-by-step example.

Protocol No. 11: a Detailed Example

1st Stage – PREPARATION

Use kinesiology (or another testing tool) to find the answers. Data thus obtained will be automatically processed by the body's innate intelligence and the genetic code's consciousness, in accordance with your intention.

*This means, for example, that if we test the level of integrity and obtain a percentage lower than 100%, or when it is necessary to get a YES and we get a NO (or vice versa), **this data is taken to be a fact and will be automatically adjusted by the reprogramming process.** WE DO NOT NEED TO KNOW THE REASON.*

Purpose of the Protocol

A client, for example, is not being considered for promotions to which he believes he is entitled.

1. **TEST if the reprogrammer (and not the person receiving the treatment) can use this protocol.**
   If YES, go immediately to Step 2.
   If NO,
   A Do not proceed with this reprogramming.
   B. Return to the preceding chapter and perform that (those) reprogramming(s) first.
   I get a YES. If all the protocols from Chapter 3 had not been done, I might have obtained a NO.

2. **A. Identify the negative emotion to be integrated into the DNA by this reprogramming.**
   B. TEST if it is the right one.
      If NO, go to Appendix IV, find another emotion and TEST if it is the right one before proceeding to Step 3.

After discussion with the client, we choose to integrate the emotion "to be scorned" in the DNA.

However, by testing, I ascertain that it is not the right emotion. I go to Appendix IV to test the list of emotions and get a YES for "bitterness." My client is indeed very bitter about this matter, as he himself admits when I tell him of the results of my search in Appendix IV. I check again if "bitterness" is the right emotion and I get a YES. If I had not found anything in Appendix IV, I could also have tested in Appendix V or let my intuition guide me to find the appropriate negative emotion.

3. **TEST if it is appropriate to install the negative magnetic charge program bound to this emotion in the DNA.**

   If NO,

   A. **Do not proceed with this reprogramming.**

   B. **TEST how much time is needed (days, weeks, months) before testing again.**

   If YES,

   A. **TEST in which chromosome** (1 to 46...) **and in which gene** (1 to 5,000+) **you must install this new program and**

   B. **TEST how many codons** (1 to 30,000+) **it comprises.**

   I get a YES.

   I find that I must integrate the negative magnetic charge linked to the emotion of "bitterness" in gene 326 of chromosome 32, and that this program contains 31 codons.

4. **TEST if this program already existed in the original divine plan of the person's DNA.**

   If YES,

   A. **TEST if it can be reproduced here.**

   B. **TEST if a bridge must be installed.**

   I get a YES.

   I can reproduce it here.

   It is not necessary to install a bridge.

5. **TEST if there is a harmful program or theme in resonance (echo) or duality (polarity) that could interfere with the new program.**

   I test each word and find that there is a harmful theme in duality with the one I am installing. I go to the next step, because this theme will be automatically included in the program.

6. **TEST if there are memories attached or linked to former programs that could interfere with integrating this new program in the DNA.**
   If YES, how many memories are there?
   I get a YES. I test to find how many memories there are and get 33. This information is automatically integrated in the reprogramming.

7. **TEST if the person can live outside the event that triggers this emotion and which provides the negative charge.**
   I get a NO. I therefore include this information in the reprogramming through my intent. The intent here is, of course, that the person have access to this magnetic charge without repeatedly needing the event (lack of promotions) that triggers the negative emotion (bitterness).

8. **TEST if the person still needs that type of event to have access to the negative charge.**
   I get a NO (my client does not need to be denied promotions to benefit from the negative magnetic charge corresponding to the emotion of "bitterness"). This means that he can now let go of that old scenario.

9. **TEST if the person can live outside of duality and integrate the two opposing forces without needing the triggering event.**
   Since human beings are used to living in duality and passing from one pole to another rather than living in a "neutral" state that remains creative even in the absence of negative events, it is important to verify this.
   I get a NO. This information is integrated automatically through intent in the reprogramming.

10. **TEST if the memory of this type of event must be placed at zero point or dissolved in all incarnations - past, present or future - and in all dimensions.**
    Since time is not linear on the energetic level, it is important to test all of the words. I test and obtain that it is necessary to dissolve the memories in all incarnations and put them at zero point in all dimensions. The reprogramming will take this into account.
    This is important so as to avoid old memories cancelling the effects of the reprogramming.

11. **TEST if the stress related to this type of event must be placed at zero point or dissolved.**
    It must be dissolved. The reprogramming will take this into account and it will be done in accordance with my intent.
    Now that my client no longer needs the triggering event, I can lighten his being by dissolving the stress accumulated on the numerous occasions when he was not considered for a promotion.

12. **TEST if all miasmas that have entered or been activated by this type of event must be placed at zero point or cancelled.**

Miasmas are voids or energetic faults that make us more vulnerable to certain pathologies or psychological imbalances. Although vibratory, miasmas can manifest themselves physically at the cellular level under certain conditions.

I do not get a YES when testing all of the words of this sentence. This means that there were no miasmas.

13. **A. TEST how many fragments have separated themselves from the person because of this type of event OR what percentage of the person is fragmented and separated because of this type of event.**

    B. TEST if it is appropriate to bring these fragments into the present at zero point and to anchor them in the DNA.

Certain traumas can provoke a fragmentation of the being that can only be complete when it has reassembled all of its fragments.

A. I find 15 fragments.

B. I find that it is appropriate; the reprogramming will take this into account aligning itself with my intention.

14. **TEST if there is a familial pattern related to this negative emotion.**
    If YES,
    - **A. TEST how many generations it goes back.**
    - **B. TEST if you must incorporate it into the DNA as a negative magnetic charge.**

In the same way that one is afraid of negative emotions before understanding that they are an important magnetic force to create with, the idea of anchoring the charge of negative familial emotional patterns inside DNA can seem daunting. However, it is by integrating it at zero point that we can put an end to the constant reactivation of familial programs.

I find that there is a familial pattern and that it goes back five generations.

15. **TEST if the negative magnetic polarity of this emotion must be installed in the following zones of conflict so that they can be at zero point:**
    A. the brain;
    B. the endocrine glands;
    C. the nervous system and the peptides;
    D. the cells, the intra and extracellular fluids, the interstitial void, the atoms and the quantum elements (quarks, muons, strands, …);
    E. the 13 helixes, chakras, etheric bodies, and the soul;
    F. another location (see Appendix III).

Conflicts can leave traces and create weak zones where energy does not circulate well. By installing the negative magnetic polarity there, we break the resistances in the conflict zones, which can then regain their strength.

I say the command out loud while testing each word. The words "cells" and "intra and extracellular fluids" test NO and that is automatically integrated in the reprogramming.

16. **TEST if the person has access to the negative charge installed by this reprogramming.**
I get a NO. My client has not yet accessed the negative charge, even though it is installed. I therefore include this information in the reprogramming so that it be adjusted in such a way that he has access to it.

17. **TEST if the person can say YES to the corresponding positive charge.**
Because, in a sense, I am installing a new route at the level of the negative polarity, I must also make sure that my client also has access to the corresponding positive charge. I get a YES.

18. **TEST if the person's genetic code contains the program to maintain the positive polarity in the presence of the negative polarity without them neutralizing each other.**
I get a NO. I include this information in the reprogramming and the desired program will be installed in his genetic code.

19. **TEST if the integration of the negative force creates a destabilization of the positive force.**
Previously, it was the positive force (yang) that dominated. Installing the negative magnetic force may create an imbalance in the well-established system.
I get a YES. This information will be integrated in the reprogramming through intent.

20. **TEST if the negative or positive force will undergo an electric or magnetic shock in this process.**
If YES,
TEST if it is necessary to install a code in the new program so that it can repolarize itself at zero point.
COMMAND its installation on chromosome __ (1 to 46...) and on gene __ (1 to 5000+), with __ codons (1 to 30,000+).
I get a YES for both "positive force" and "electric or magnetic shock." The newly inserted negative force in my client's DNA must make a place for itself next to the positive force already present. Like all sudden change, this challenge causes a shock.
I also test that the new program will have to include a code for the positive force to repolarize itself. This information is now part of the reprogramming.

21. **TEST if the person was giving the negative magnetic charge generated by this emotion to another entity.**
    If YES,
    A. TEST which percentage of this energy was thus given.
    B.   TEST if there was an alliance on this subject with this entity. If YES, put it at zero point or dissolve it.
    I get a YES. Nothing is lost, nothing is created. Since my client was not using the negative magnetic force generated by the emotion of "bitterness," it was used elsewhere.
    I test to find the percentage and I get 76%. There was an alliance and I test that it must be dissolved. Consequently, my client will be able to reappropriate at 100% the negative charge of the emotion of "bitterness".

22. **TEST if the person can come to manifest events at 100% without needing a difficult emotion to generate the necessary negative magnetic force.**
    I get a YES. This means that the power of my client to manifest positive events at 100% does not depend anymore on an event generating the emotion of "bitterness".

23. **TEST if the person can integrate the new negative charge into his/her daily life.**
    I test NO. This information is included automatically in the reprogramming to make sure that the new negative force be well integrated in his daily life for it to be truly efficient.

24. **TEST if it is necessary to install a bridge between the physical body and the negative magnetic charge.**
    I get a YES. This means that the body has efficiently recorded the magnetic change.

25. **TEST if the integration of the negative force is at zero point.**
    I test NO. This information is included automatically in the reprogramming to make sure that the integration be at zero point.

26. **TEST if it is necessary to enter other data in this program before installing the program.** If YES, go to Appendix III and follow the instructions to test which data must be entered in this reprogramming. Then, return to the protocol and proceed to the next stage.
    I obtain NO. I therefore go to the Installation Stage.

    The second part of the protocol is the installation. It is the same as for all previous protocols.

Johanne S. sent me an eloquent testimony about this protocol.

I was so enthusiastic about the integration technique that I wanted everyone around me to benefit from this revolutionary method. Therefore I slowly began the therapeutic process by mentioning to people that, although we were embarking on a journey that would lead us to a destination, we did not know whether our innate intelligence would take us on a side road, a country road, a bumpy road in bad need of repair or a speedway. Our innate intelligence would be our guide. Our purpose was to find the main emotional theme [the core issue] which had been omnipresent throughout our long passage here on Earth. I put myself at zero point and allowed for guidance. Following some discussions and an exchange of ideas, we would be able to conclude and define the "negative charge" that needed to be integrated in a short 20 to 25 minute session.

The results were extraordinary. I received feedback from the people I had treated and I could verify with them the changes that had occurred following the treatment. Furthermore, after having treated women intensely for two months, I inevitably realized that I was also including myself and that this experience had allowed me to discover my own recurrent emotional theme.

I am now able to receive from life what is best for me: abundance and prosperity in all good things on the frequency of love at zero point.

Another client brought to my attention that, after including the magnetic charge of incest into her genetic code, she fell into a deep silence. She mentioned that before doing the protocol she always felt a buzzing mechanical tension inside her body. Upon installation of Protocol 11, this clenching sensation immediately stopped and never returned.

PROTOCOL NO. 12

Integrating the Positive Polarity

When I began integrating the magnetic charge of my negative emotions, I started to feel a new sense of power inside of me. I felt strong but without an ego, a totally new sensation in my life, a true sense of well-being.

Then, one day, as I was driving my car on my way to lunch with my father, I had another amazing inspirational moment. I told myself that if people were put on this Earth to test out emotions and incorporate their charge, then perhaps we could acquire power without it being continuously triggered by difficult situations. How amazing it would be if we could also have access to the positive charge of happy moments without necessarily having to relive them constantly. In other words, why not develop a protocol that would allow us to integrate the positive charges? After all, when you stop to think about it, we also tend to shop for happy moments to then let the charge go and start all over again without harvesting it. Wouldn't it be great to have access to the positive polarity of a trip to the Pacific Islands, a wonderful surprise, or any other event that stimulates our positive polarities without having to take a vacation or wait for our spouse to surprise us?

So I went ahead and developed the protocol. Since I began working with this new protocol, I have discovered new things, as you, yourself, will surely do. For example, I integrated into my genetic code the pleasure, the passion, the mystery, the excitement and the happiness which had been provided by an old lingering love whose memory refused to disappear from my life. I kept hidden inside my heart this beautiful story that ended badly. The regret had never subsided even though I had begun a new life, and a good one at that, with someone else. Therefore, to be able to access those positive charges when I needed them, I installed the positive qualities of that romantic experience inside my DNA. Now that I carry this beauty inside myself, I feel liberated from this old story and I managed to get closure of this issue without any regrets. In fact, I feel like I have blossomed from this!

You can use this protocol to install whatever state you wish: a state of bliss, security, freedom and so on. I thought I would suggest, at this point, a short list of positive charges to integrate into your DNA. As a possibility, you may integrate a positive charge that is familiar to you, like the ones mentioned previously for example, or you can test the suggestions in the list below to see if one is appropriate for you at this time.

1. OM AHIMSA AHIMSA OM (the peace mantra)
2. AUM MANE PADME OM (The "Heart of the Lotus" is the compassion mantra used by Buddhists who study with the Dalai Lama.)
3. NAM MYOHO RENGE KYO (The principle of simultaneity of cause and effect or the instant manifestation of the results of prayer.)
4. OM NAMAH SHIVAYA (This is a very powerful mantra that brings light.)
5. LOVE OF SELF
6. I AM GOD/GODDESS.
7. ASCENSION
8. ENCOURAGEMENT
9. WE SHALL OVERCOME. (or "This time, we will overcome this.")
10. SOUL MATE (I have a soul mate who is currently here on Earth; my mate is available and accessible.)
11. ABUNDANCE (financial, sexual, emotional, spiritual, mental, stellar or other)
12. SUCCESS
13. BLISS
14. FRIENDSHIP/LOVE

I therefore invite you to have some fun with Protocol 12. Incorporate the positive charges into your DNA and use the integrated polarity to regenerate your health.

PROTOCOL NO. 12

Integrating the Positive Polarity

This protocol is very similar to Protocol 11, however, it was designed to integrate positive charges. We can, for example, include in the DNA a positive charge such as: "There exists, on this Earth, a soul mate just for me." We can also inscribe the positive charge of happy events for which we would like to benefit without needing to re-experience. For example, we can integrate the positive charge "relaxing vacation" and continuously benefit from this charge without being on vacation all the time. Another example is one that relates to romantic relationships. If we are having trouble letting go of a happy love affair that has ended, we can integrate a positive charge such as "pleasure" or "being loved" and have access to feelings (and energies) of happiness that it brought to us without having to constantly remember the person or the times spent together.

1ˢᵗ Stage of Protocol	**1ˢᵗ Stage – PREPARATION**
Identifies the object of the protocol as well as the data to be included in the reprogramming process.	Before beginning to test, set your intent by saying: ***I choose to be at zero point even if I don't know how***. Use kinesiology (or another testing tool) to find the answers. Data thus obtained will be automatically processed by the body's innate intelligence and the genetic code's consciousness, in accordance with your intention.

This test is important.	1. **TEST if the reprogrammer (not the person receiving the treatment) can use this protocol.**
	If YES, go immediately to Step 2.
	If NO,
	    A. **Do not proceed with this reprogramming.**
	    B. **Return to the preceding chapter and perform that (those) reprogramming(s) first.**

The precise emotion is the one to integrate as the positive magnetic charge in the DNA in order to reach the objective. For example: a person who wishes to end financial problems could believe that the positive emotional charge to be installed is "feeling rich" although we must integrate "independence" or "freedom", etc.

2. A. **Identify the positive emotion to be integrated into the DNA by this reprogramming.**
   B. **TEST if it is the right one.**
      If NO, go to Appendix V (New Structure) or to the previous page, find another emotion and TEST if it is the right one before proceeding to Step 3.

We may obtain a NO for several reasons. We don't need to know why. Simply respect this information.

Finding the exact DNA address is the MAIN PIVOT of all reprogramming. In general, the program is in one gene of a single chromosome.

3. **TEST if it is appropriate to install the positive magnetic charge program bound to this emotion in the DNA.**
   If NO,
      A. **Do not perform this reprogramming.**
      B. **TEST how much time is needed (days, weeks, months) before testing again.**
   If YES,
      A. **TEST in which chromosome** (1 to 46…) **and in which gene** (1 to 5,000+) **you must install this new program and**
      B. **TEST how many codons** (1 to 30,000+) **it comprises.**

The original DNA plan is the underlying diagram that precedes all genetic mutation. If this information still exists in a latent form, it will automatically be included in the reprogramming.

4. **TEST if the program already existed in the original divine plan of the person's DNA.**
   If YES,
      A. **TEST if it can be reproduced here.**
      B. **TEST if a bridge must be installed.**

A theme or another program may neutralize the installation of the new program.

5. TEST if there is a harmful program or theme in resonance (echo) or duality (polarity) that could interfere with the new program.

Memories of former programs are capable of interfering with the new program.

**6. TEST if there are memories attached or linked to former programs that could interfere with the reconnection of this new program in the DNA.
If YES, how many are there?**

The answer must be NO. If it isn't, this data will automatically be included in the reprogramming.

7. TEST if the person still needs the event that triggers this emotion to have access to the positive charge.

8. TEST if you can recuperate, reintegrate and reactivate the memory of this type of event in all incarnations - past, present or future - and in all dimensions.

9. TEST if you must integrate the well being related to this kind of event in the DNA.

Refer to Appendix II on how to test a number.

**10. TEST if there is a familial pattern related to this positive emotion.
If YES,**
　　A. TEST how many generations it goes back.
　　B. TEST if you must incorporate it into the DNA as a positive magnetic charge.

The answer must be YES. If it isn't, this data will automatically be included in the reprogramming.

11. TEST if the endorphins are rebalanced by this program.

12. TEST if the person being treated has access to the positive charge installed by this reprogramming.

If you need to identify the emotion, refer to Appendix IV.

13. TEST if the person can say YES to the corresponding negative charge. Is it important to know which one?

We must get a NO. This data will be automatically included in the reprogramming.

14. TEST if the integration of the positive force creates a destabilization of the negative force.

Test each word.

15. TEST if the negative or positive force will undergo an electric or magnetic shock in this process.
If YES,
    TEST if a code must be installed to allow the new program to repolarize itself at zero point.
    COMMAND its installation in chromosome (1 to 46...) **and in gene** (1 to 5000+), **with** (1 to 30,000+) **codons.**

16. TEST if the person can live outside duality and integrate the two opposing forces without needing the triggering event.

17. TEST if the integration of the positive charge is at zero point.

Just as nothing is lost and nothing is created, the positive charges that we do not integrate can be used by other entities. Test if the charge must be put at zero point or dissolved.

18. TEST if the person was giving the positive magnetic charge generated by this emotion to another entity.
If YES,
    A. TEST which percentage of this energy was thus given.
    B. TEST if there was an alliance on this subject with this entity. If YES, put it at zero point or dissolve it.

19. TEST if the person can come to manifest events at 100% without needing a happy moment or event to generate the positive magnetic force necessary.

20. TEST if the person can integrate the new positive charge into his/her daily life.

We may have felt an emotion and integrated it in the genetic code without the body's knowledge.

21. TEST if it is necessary to install a bridge between the physical body and the positive magnetic charge.

22. TEST if it is necessary to cancel or put at zero point the miasmas that entered or were activated by this type of event.

23. TEST if the person's genetic code contains the program permitting him/her to maintain the positive polarity in the presence of the negative polarity without them neutralizing each other.

24. TEST if the positive charge can exist in the darkness.

Before installing the program, it may be necessary to input other data.

25. TEST if it is necessary to enter other data in this program before its installation. If YES, go to Appendix III and follow the instructions to test which data must be entered in this reprogramming. Then, return to the protocol and proceed to the next stage.

2nd Stage – The installation takes into account all the data found in the first stage. Insofar as the command is spoken out loud, each item is integrated in the reprogramming. Please use the tone of voice you would use for a prayer or hypnosis as the DNA responds to language spoken in this fashion.

2nd Stage – INSTALLATION OF THE REPROGRAMMING

1. SAY: *I COMMAND that this new program be installed in the nucleus of the master cell of the pineal gland in all lives and all dimensions.*

2. SAY: *I COMMAND that, from the pineal gland, this program reach:*
   A. *the endocrine glands;*
   B. *the brain, the nervous system and the peptides;*
   C. *the cells, the intra and extracellular fluids, the interstitial void, the atoms and the quantum elements (quarks, muons, strands, …);*
   D. *all of the helixes, chakras, etheric bodies, and the soul;*
   E. *another location* (see Appendix III).

If Point E tests YES , refer to Appendix III and find the area.

3. SAY: *I COMMAND the RNA to support and reconnect itself to this new program.*

The original DNA plan is the underlying pattern that precedes all genetic mutation.

4. **SAY: *I COMMAND* the codons to return to the order of the perfect original program even if there has been an inversion of codes.**

5. **SAY: *I COMMAND* the speed of the photons and the structure of the DNA spiral to adjust themselves.**

6. **SAY: *I COMMAND* that the connection within the corpus callosum of the brain be restored according to the original divine plan.**

The telomere is part of the very structure of the chromosome. It is a protein found at the ends of the chromosomal strands in DNA that protects these strands. In simpler terms, it is the end of each chromosome. The telomerase is an enzyme that acts as the "glue" of the telomere.

7. **SAY: *I COMMAND* the perfect integrity of the telomere and the telomerase.**

Refer to Appendix VII for a list of systems.

8. **SAY: *I COMMAND* that any residues from old programs be eliminated through the appropriate systems.**

9. **SAY: *I COMMAND* that this program be perfectly sealed.**

Refer to Appendix I for the definition of Merkabah.

10. **SAY: *I COMMAND* that the Merkabah be perfectly sealed.**

11. **SAY: *I COMMAND* that no radiation affect the DNA or RNA.**

12. **SAY: *I COMMAND* that this new program be installed completely, and until further notice, in the brain stem, here and now.**

13. **SAY: *I COMMAND* that the reconnection of this new program be perfectly tolerated and integrated and that this occurs at zero point.**

ESSENTIAL POINT
in reprogramming

14. SAY: *I COMMAND that the power, the harmony and the purity of this new program be installed in the DNA and be perfectly activated.*

3rd Stage

3rd Stage – CONCLUSION OF THE PROTOCOL

The installation of other data may be required before concluding the protocol.

15. TEST if it is necessary to include other data in the reprogramming for it to be effective, tolerated or integrated. If YES, go to Appendix III and follow the instructions to test which data must be entered in this reprogramming. Then, return to the protocol and proceed to Step 16.

This closes the protocol.

16. SAY: *I COMMAND that this reprogramming be tolerated and integrated, according to the original divine plan, in the frequency of love, even if our helixes have been deactivated in the past.*

This seals the reprogramming.

17. SAY: *I COMMAND that this regeneration be complete and sealed, until further notice from … (the person being reprogrammed).*

Whether we use Protocol 11 to integrate the negative polarity or Protocol 12 to integrate the positive polarity, we are taking a big step on our evolutionary path. Our soul searches for experiences to accumulate. It is one of the reasons for our existence here on Earth. By integrating emotions and experiences into our genetic code, we work to help our soul to achieve richness and to enhance its past existences. Wisdom will be imparted without needing to trigger positive or negative events.

Incorporating the magnetic charges of our past experiences also increases our magnetic power so that once our commands are stated, they have greater impact. Let us take as an example the case of one of my students who chose to integrate "professional success" into her DNA. This woman is an accountant who does consulting work for businesses. Her profession constantly requires her to rebuild companies that are in critical positions. She no sooner finishes one case when she is onto the next. Everywhere she goes she is able to rebuild the team spirit of the groups that she works with. She is so rich with positive experiences that by inserting the feeling of success into her genetic code, she increases not only her positive magnetic charge, but also her magnetic power when she wants to be successful in other areas.

In the past few years, astronomers have observed a new big bang from which they figure that a new universe has been born. Certain sources (see Appendix VIII) have stated that this universe is populated by beings who know how to integrate feminine and masculine, positive and negative polarities at zero point. However, in order to integrate these two forces, it is essential to know them. This is what being human truly means and we are currently evolving towards the integration of these two forces. Nobody can deny that negative and positive polarities belong to our third dimension. We, humans, are undoubtedly the experts in the field of emotional charges. Can you name a person who has never experienced moodiness, sadness, joy or happiness? We are able to vibrate within duality. Our error lies in the belief that it is a weakness rather than a gift. By escaping our uncomfortable feelings, we bypass our wealth. And, since it is here, on Earth, that we live and feel negative charges, it therefore means that it is from here, from our universe, that we will create by uniting both these polarities.

When we balance both polarities within us, we are automatically in a state of compassion and love. If we are able to integrate the negative and positive charges of our past, we will automatically create what we want in a balanced and harmonious way. Since we already carry a wide range of experiences in the field of unbalanced polarities, I believe that we are now ready to integrate this experience and create a new reality in a state of love at zero point, rather than with the polarized energy of the positive or the negative.

Chapter 5

HOW DO WE LIVE WITH
OUR NEW PROGRAMS?

N ow that the dormant part of us has awakened and is taking over the reprogramming of its genetic codes, we will continue to install new programs
throughout our life. This will help us become sovereign, free, happy,
wealthy, secure and live a life of abundance. In this chapter, we will take a look at
new possibilities currently accessible through our new programs.

PROTOCOL NO. 13

Living in the Moment

To be able to live comfortably with the change of frequency innate to reprogramming, we must be able to keep our attention focused on living in the moment.

When we talked about our programs by default in Chapter 2, there was an
aspect that we did not explore; the "transfer of the by-default intention", also
referred to as the "trance." The mention of the term "transfer" here applies to the
transfer of a past situation into our current reality, which causes it to be biased and
faulty. We fall into a trance, which brings us back to our childhood years, for example, even if we are 30, 45, 50 or older. All our reactions and feelings often belong to
the past, not to our current reality. I have often noticed that when we do not feel
good, the reason often has something to do with the past and nothing to do with
the current moment. It may be a heaviness that belongs to our childhood or a
future plan that seems to slip through our fingers.

The first time I became aware of transferring unconscious intention from our childhood or trance phenomenon, I prayed that, when I fell for it, I would be able to recognize this unconsciously repeating program from the past, and put it to rest. In fact, there are all kinds of small signs that tell me that I am not in the present but back in childhood. Over time, I have been able to become aware of them. They include the feeling of being closed in and powerless, a certain tone of voice, posture, breathing amplitude, internal doubt, etc. All those elements have made me more aware of the necessity of putting together a process to stop the transfer and end the trance because it takes us away from the current moment.

Our programs by default can also bring us into the future. For example, I start to worry about my plans for the autumn even if I am only at the end of spring. The irises have just started to bloom and I am already concerned that September will not be a good month! How is it that we look to the future rather than live in the present? It is because of an overload due to a former program intense enough to dissociate or make us leave our bodies (remember that many of us learned this when we were children). This program by default can be of emotional, mental, physical or spiritual nature. It is important to note that when we leave our bodies, we lose power, because the connection to our vital energy is lost. For this reason, the energy no longer circulates as it should.

There is still another force, which we have yet to speak of, that prevents us from living in the moment and destroys our means and energies. The moment has come for me to bring up the subject.

According to several authors, there could have been, at the beginning of creation, a force that refused to move forward and incarnate. It is called the "anti-creation regressive force" and is opposed to the movement of creation. However, we are not forced to surrender our vital force to this anti-creation movement because of the law of free will. Nevertheless, it can happen that at certain points in our life we become depressed and no longer want to participate in the creative movement. We can slowly fall into the frequencies of the anti-creation regressive force, and if we let ourselves go and willingly abandon our vital energy in that way, the regressive anti-creation force wins us over. In order to be 100% present and participate in the creative process, we must repossess that part of ourselves. This is the reason for Protocol 13, whose main objective is to help us stay completely in the present, at zero point.

Without further ado, I invite you to get familiar with Protocol 13.

PROTOCOL NO. 13

Living in the Present at Zero Point

1st Stage of Protocol

Identifies the object of the protocol as well as the data to be included in the reprogramming process.

1st Stage – PREPARATION

Before beginning to test, set your intent by saying: *I choose to be at zero point even if I don't know how.*

Use kinesiology (or another testing tool) to find the answers. Data thus obtained will be automatically processed by the body's innate intelligence and the genetic code's consciousness, in accordance with your intention.

To find the particular situation, ask the person questions or, in case of doubt, test in Appendix III.

1. **TEST if the person can live completely in the present at zero point.**
   A. in general, OR
   B. in regard to a particular situation to be included in this session.
      If YES,
         TEST which specific situation.

To test if a person can affirm something, ask him/her to say this sentence out loud. (Ex.: "It is normal for me to be at zero point.") Test while the person is speaking.

2. **TEST if the person can affirm that it is normal to live in the present at zero point in general or in regard to this situation.**

We may obtain a NO for several reasons. We don't need to know why. Simply respect this information.

3. **TEST if it is appropriate to install a program to be completely in the present at zero point in the DNA.**
   If NO,
      A. Do not perform this reprogramming.
      B. TEST how much time is needed (days, weeks, months) before testing again.

Finding the exact DNA address is the MAIN PIVOT of all reprogramming. In general, the program is in one gene of a single chromosome.

If YES,

   A. **TEST in which chromosome** (1 to 46...) **and in which gene** (1 to 5,000+) **this new program must be installed and**

   B. **TEST how many codons** (1 to 30,000+) **it comprises.**

The original DNA plan is the underlying diagram that precedes all genetic mutation. If this information still exists in a latent form, it will automatically be included in the reprogramming.

4. **TEST if the program already existed in the original divine plan of the person's DNA.**
   If YES,
   A. **TEST if it can be reproduced here.**
   B. **TEST if a bridge must be installed.**

A theme or another program may neutralize the installation of the new program.

5. **TEST if there is a harmful program or theme in resonance (echo) or duality (polarity) that could interfere with the new program.**

Memories of former programs are capable of interfering with the new program.

6. **TEST if there are memories attached or linked to former programs that could interfere with the reconnection of this new program in the DNA.**
   If YES, how many are there?

The answer must be YES. If it isn't, this data will be automatically included in the reprogramming.

7. **TEST if the person can put the past or the future at zero point.**

Always test each word when verifying.

Refer to Appendix II on how to test a number.

8. **TEST if a part of the person is living in the past or the future.**
   If YES,
   A. **TEST how many fragments are involved OR the percentage of the person that is living in the past or the future.**

There could be hun-dreds, even thousands, of fragments.

B. **TEST if it is appropriate to bring these fragments into the present at zero point and to anchor them in the DNA.**

Ask he/she to say it out loud and test while he/she is speaking.

9. **TEST if the person can assert that he/she chooses to live 100% in the present with his/her 13 helixes.**

Refer to Appendix II on how to test a number.

10.**A.** **TEST which percentage of the person's karma remains linked to the past or the future.**
   B. **TEST if it must be put at zero point or dissolved.**

Ask the person to repeat this affirmation out loud and test while he/she is speaking.

11. **TEST if the person knows that he/she can let go of the past or the future and live in the present, while being loved by others.**

At the beginning of Appendix III, we explain how to test to find the information.

12. **TEST if something is blocking the person from living in the present in the new frequency with his/her 13 helixes.**

The answer must be NO. If it isn't, this data will automatically be included in the reprogramming.

13. **TEST if the person is stuck in the no-time and/or the no-space.**

The answer must be YES. If it isn't, this data will automatically be included in the reprogramming.

14. **TEST if his/her roots are 100% in the present and in the right location.**

We could be anchored elsewhere. They must be in the present.

15. **TEST if his/her emotions or expectations (emotional or mental) are anchored in the present, past or future.**

Test each word.

16. **TEST if his/her intents, when he/she formulates them, are bound to the present, past or future.**

17. **TEST if there is a familial pattern that holds the person in the past or in the future.**
If YES,
 A. **TEST how many generations it goes back to.**
 B. **TEST if it must be put at zero point or dissolved.**

Example: marriage, vows of fidelity, religious vows, etc.

18. **TEST if there are alliances or vows that bind the person to the past or the future.**
If YES,
 TEST if they must be put at zero point or dissolved.

Test each word. Courses, initiations, energy work, etc. could have had a positive impact when they were done and yet become a source of imbalance in the present.

19. **TEST if there is a course, a form of training or meditation, an initiation (shamanic or other), or energy therapy or another activity or intervention of this nature, in the past, the present or the future that:**
 A. **bind(s) the person to the past or projects him/her into the future OR**
 B. **create(s) an imbalance.**
 If YES,
 TEST if it (they) must be put at zero point or dissolved.

We must get a YES for each element tested. If the opposite occurs, this data will be automatically included in the reprogramming.

20.A. **TEST if the energies, helixes, chakras, etheric bodies and the soul of the person are perfectly sealed in the present.**
 B. **TEST if another part or element of the person is not 100% in the present.**

21. **TEST if a rivalry between the frequencies of the present, past and future keeps the person in the past or future.**

22. **TEST if a faulty program or concept, in the past, present or future, prevents the person from living completely in the present.**

Every time we use or put into action a creative force that is not at zero point, it can generate the opposite polarity – meaning the "anti-creation regressive force."

23. A. TEST if a part of the person's vital energy has yielded to the regressive anti-creation force. If YES,
> **A. TEST the percentage which has yielded.**
> **B. TEST if it can be completely recuperated. If not, test how much (percentage) can be recuperated at this moment.**

B. TEST if there is an anchorage in the regressive anti-creation force. If YES,
> **TEST if it must be put at zero point or dissolved.**

C. TEST if the person needs a bridge or a link to get out of the regressive anti-creation force.

Before installing the program, it may be necessary to input other data.

24. TEST if it is necessary to enter other data in this program before its installation. If YES, go to Appendix III and follow the instructions to test which data must be entered in this reprogramming. Then, return to the protocol and proceed to the next stage.

2nd Stage – The installation takes into account all the data found in the first stage.

2nd Stage – INSTALLATION OF THE REPROGRAMMING

Insofar as the command is spoken out loud, each item is integrated in the reprogramming. Please use the tone of voice you would use for a prayer or hypnosis as the DNA responds to language spoken in this fashion.

1. SAY: *I COMMAND that this new program be installed in the nucleus of the master cell of the pineal gland in all lives and all dimensions.*

2. SAY: *I COMMAND that, from the pineal gland, this program reach:*
A. *the endocrine glands;*
B. *the brain, the nervous system and the peptides;*
C. *the cells, the intra and extracellular fluids, the interstitial void, the atoms and the quantum elements (quarks, muons, strands, …);*
D. *all of the helixes, chakras, etheric bodies, and the soul;*
E. *another location* (see Appendix III).

If Point E tests YES, refer to Appendix III and find the area.

3. **SAY: *I COMMAND the RNA to support and reconnect itself to this new program.***

The original DNA plan is the underlying pattern that precedes all genetic mutation.

4. **SAY: *I COMMAND the codons to return to the order of the perfect original program even if there has been an inversion of codes.***

5. **SAY: *I COMMAND the speed of the photons and the structure of the DNA spiral to adjust themselves.***

6. **SAY: *I COMMAND that the connection within the corpus callosum of the brain be restored according to the original divine plan.***

The telomere is part of the very structure of the chromosome. It is a protein found at the ends of the chromosomal strands in DNA that protects these strands. In simpler terms, it is the end of each chromosome. The telomerase is an enzyme that acts as the "glue" of the telomere.

7. **SAY: *I COMMAND the perfect integrity of the telomere and the telomerase.***

Refer to Appendix VII for a list of systems.

8. **SAY: *I COMMAND that any residues from old programs be eliminated through the appropriate systems.***

9. **SAY: *I COMMAND that this program be perfectly sealed.***

Refer to Appendix I for the definition of Merkabah.

10. **SAY: *I COMMAND that the Merkabah be perfectly sealed.***

11. **SAY: *I COMMAND that no radiation affect the DNA or RNA.***

12. **SAY: *I COMMAND that this new program be installed completely, and until further notice, in the brain stem, here and now.***

13. SAY: *I COMMAND that the reconnection of this new program be perfectly tolerated and integrated and that this occurs at zero point.*

ESSENTIAL POINT in reprogramming

14. SAY: *I COMMAND that the power, the harmony and the purity of this new program be installed in the DNA and be perfectly activated.*

3rd Stage

3rd Stage – CONCLUSION OF THE PROTOCOL

The installation of other data may be required before concluding the protocol.

15. TEST if it is necessary to include other data in the reprogramming for it to be effective, tolerated or integrated. If YES, go to Appendix III and follow the instructions to test which data must be entered in this reprogramming. Then, return to the protocol and proceed to Step 16.

This closes the protocol.

16. SAY: *I COMMAND that this reprogramming be tolerated and integrated, according to the original divine plan, in the frequency of love, even if our helixes have been deactivated in the past.*

This seals the reprogramming.

17. SAY: *I COMMAND that this regeneration be complete and sealed, until further notice from ... (the person being reprogrammed).*

The 13 Allies Within

I always felt a sense of relief when I was reminded by reading or from others that I was not alone, that I was being guided. I had never seen my allies however, and was not aware of their names until a third person provided me with the information. I knew that there was synchronicity in my life and, although difficult at times, I felt in my heart that my path was established and orderly. Yet I still wondered who or what always gave me the strength that I needed? Was it my passion, my courage or my allies? I had no idea.

At one point, before I started to work with DNA, I decided, since I did not clearly hear my allies, to take the bull by the horns and co-create with God/Goddess within in order to obtain what I needed. In other words, I stopped waiting for my allies to save me and tell me what I should do regarding my health or other issues. With this action, I broke the cycle of wishful thinking. Without realizing it, I had just chosen to co-create what I needed and to regain sovereignty over my DNA.

Once I began my work on DNA, I heard my inner voice more clearly. Surprisingly, it was only later, after I had activated my 13 helixes that I contacted my allies! They introduced themselves as vibratory allies that were linked to the 13 helixes within. If you suppose that this was revealed to me during deep meditation in a zen center by the ocean, think again! It happened while eating a pizza with two of my best friends. At one point, all three of us realized simultaneously that each and every helix in our body was connected to an ally.

Our helixes were not only connected to our chakras, but also to our allies, co-creators, messengers and intergalactic relays. From that moment on, I did not need to pray, search for my personal allies or my tribe, find where I fit in the big picture, or establish contact with the universe. I knew that the answer vibrated in the heart of each and every cell within the spirals of my DNA.

When we live with only two helixes and life is but a series of events influenced by the polarizations of duality, we are constantly torn between the guardian angel on one side and the devil on the other. Once we repossess our genetic code and choose to live out of the polarized duality, we must reshuffle our guardian angels, who are no longer the guides of light protecting us from the guides of darkness that scare us. This reshuffling happens, if you wish, when we choose to live with 13 allies who co-create with us at zero point. On that note, I would like to introduce, in the following chart, my 13 allies.

As you will see, the 13 allies are not polarized. Because they are always in the state of love at zero point, where Light meets Darkness, and because they are connected to our 13 helixes, there is no doubt that we have the power and the capacity to co-create with them a non-linear reality. We are born to live in the frequency of love where polarities coexist. But before that can happen, we must install in our DNA the appropriate code that will allow us to contact our 13 allies.

By re-connecting our 13 helixes, we are able to establish contact with infinity through the infinitesimally small code tucked away inside our bodies called DNA. Protocol 13 installs in our DNA a code which allows us to easily and smoothly contact the allies within us (rather than the ones outside of us like in the sky or in a distant universe). Once our 13 allies are reconnected, all flows as if we had, in our cells, an "address" (one for each ally) through which it becomes easier to connect and communicate with them. When you have finished the following protocol, I invite you to contact one of your allies (test to make sure of your ally's presence) and ask this ally to manifest him/herself every time you want to realize an intention. I look forward to hearing from you about this.

TABLE OF THE 13 ALLIES

Ally for Helix 1	The ally of the first helix is in contact with the planet Earth. It understands the change in the seasons and our intrinsic or natural needs. This ally can help us with everything which concerns our physical health, especially the nervous system, which can be very important to some people.
Ally for Helix 2	The ally of the second helix is an adventurous creator. It is innovative, passionate and brilliant. It is our personal Einstein riding a purebred horse.
Ally for Helix 3	The ally of the third helix resembles a stream of water. Always in movement, it helps us remain fluid through emotional conflicts. It can help us resolve conflicts and establish healthy boundaries.
Ally for Helix 4	On the fourth helix, we find an ambassador directly linked to the heart of creation. It is from here that we can draw the determination to install the state of love at zero point in all that we do.
Ally for Helix 5	On the fifth helix, we find sounds and geometric shapes. This ally gives us access to geometry codes. It is from here that the protocols of DNA engineering, published in this book, are generated.
Ally for Helix 6	The ally of the sixth helix announces the new paradigm, the new vision of Ascension. Imagine Christ ascending on his cloud.
Ally for Helix 7	The ally of the seventh helix is a source of peace. Picture snow falling quietly in the countryside, in the heart of the forest where the only sounds are those of chickadees and where large pine trees soar upwards. You recognize this ally by a deep feeling of peacefulness.
Ally for Helix 8	The ally of the eighth helix is like a sphere of energy, or better, like an envelope or a vessel (Merkabah) of energy. This envelope connects us to the different corners of the planet, despite the different time zones and seasons. With this vessel, we feel connected to the entire human race.
Ally for Helix 9	The ally of the ninth helix lifts the veil over other worlds. It resembles a multicolored bridge. This ally allows us to sense the connection with our central soul and all its manifestations throughout the universe. It is the access code to all that we are and all that is not of this planet.
Ally for Helix 10	The ally of the tenth helix is our personal ambassador in the intergalactic worlds which are concerned with the preservation of the Earth.
Ally for Helix 11	The ally of the eleventh helix provides access to zero point. In a conflict situation, we call upon this ally. It then acts similar to a whirlwind that goes in all directions and puts the situation at zero point. In this state, it is not situated between the left or the right, nor between the top or the bottom. It literally becomes a point of energy that follows all kinds of sinuous curves to finally stop at a precise, center point. The situation is then at zero point and the conflict is solved. The trajectory of the point, and its path to arrive at zero point are unpredictable and different every time. In this respect, zero point is not in the middle of a sphere. It is a random point of energy. This is why zero point cannot be defined as the point at the center of duality. The eleventh helix is connected to all these dimensions and includes all these positions. It is multidirectional.
Ally for Helix 12	The "ally" of the twelfth helix is like a prayer to the Creative Power, and thus can be pictured as two hands in prayer. It is not so much an ally as it is the secret to an intimate, personal relationship between our soul and the Source of creation. We do not disturb the Source to help us cure a cold, but we do appeal to it in moments of profound reverence.
Ally for Helix 13	The ally of the thirteenth helix is a dark, black envelope, like a cocoon that envelops us in darkness. This is a comfortable and assuring darkness similar to the one experienced within the womb. This ally brings us to the world of the Shadows.

PROTOCOL NO. 14

Reconnecting the DNA with the Allies of the 13 Helixes

1ˢᵗ Stage of Protocol

Identifies the object of the protocol as well as the data to be included in the reprogramming process.

1ˢᵗ Stage – PREPARATION

Before beginning to test, set your intent by saying: *I choose to be at zero point even if I don't know how.*

Use kinesiology (or another testing tool) to find the answers. Data thus obtained will be automatically processed by the body's innate intelligence and the genetic code's consciousness, in accordance with your intention.

1. A. **TEST with how many allies you must re-establish a reconnection.**
    B. **TEST which one(s) (1 to 13).**
    C. **TEST if it is in general, OR**
    D. **in regard to a particular situation to be included in this session.**
        IF YES,
        TEST which specific situation.

We may obtain a NO for several reasons. We don't need to know why. Simply respect this information.

2. **For each ally with which you are re-establishing a connection, TEST if a program must be installed in the DNA in relation to this reconnection.**
    If NO,
    A. **Do not perform this reprogramming.**
    B. **TEST how much time is needed (days, weeks, months) before testing again.**

Finding the exact DNA address is the MAIN PIVOT of all reprogramming. In general, the program is in one gene of a single chromosome.

    If YES,
    A. **TEST in which chromosome** (1 to 46…) **and in which gene** (1 to 5,000+).
    B. **TEST how many codons** (1 to 30,000+) **are in this new program.**

3. **TEST if the ally/allies ____ communicate(s) with all the person's etheric bodies and chakras.**

Test each word of the description and include in the reprogramming those that test YES.

4. TEST the description of the ally/allies _____ . (Refer to the Table of the 13 Allies on page 172.)

Check each point for each ally with whom you re-establish a connection. If you get a YES for Point F, include another intention here. To find it, go to Annex V and test which intention it is.

5. TEST if it is necessary to install a program to better:
A. hear ally/allies No(s). _____
B. connect with ally/allies No(s). _____
C. communicate with ally/allies No(s). _____
D. be in contact with ally/allies No(s). _____
E. maintain contact with ally/allies No(s). _____
F. other intent(s) with ally/allies No(s). _____

We must get a YES. With this new program the person will end a long period of isolation and separation.

6. TEST if the person can live beyond isolation and separation while having the ally/allies within his/her genetic code.

The answer must be NO. If it isn't, this data will be automatically included in the reprogramming.

7. TEST if the person is attached to isolation and separation.

The answer must be YES.

8. TEST if the person can apply the information received from the ally/allies in his/her daily life.

We must get a YES for each ally with which we are re-establishing a connection.

9. TEST if the person can communicate with ally/allies _____ consciously.

We must get a YES for Nos. 10 and 11 for each ally tested.

10. TEST if the person can feel supported by ally/allies _____ .

11. TEST if the person can co-create with ally/allies _____ .

Test each word.

12. TEST if it is necessary to dissolve, or put at zero point the memory of the separation with ally/allies _____ in all incarnations (past, present, future) and dimensions.

13. TEST if the feeling of being lost in the universe that was caused by the separation with ally/allies ____ should be put at zero point or to cancelled.

14. TEST if it is necessary to cancel or put at zero point the miasmas that entered or were activated by the isolation and separation.

Refer to Appendix II to know how to test.

15. A. TEST how many fragments were separated from the person because of the isolation and separation OR the percentage of the person that was fragmented for this reason.
    B. TEST if it is appropriate to bring these fragments back into the present at zero point and to anchor them in the DNA.

16. For each ally with whom you re-establish a reconnection with, TEST if the person's genetic code contains the program that allows him/her to maintain contact with that ally.

The original DNA plan is the underlying diagram that precedes all genetic mutation. If this information still exists in a latent form, it will automatically be included in the reprogramming.

17. TEST if any programs installed in this protocol already existed in the original divine plan of the person's DNA. If YES,
    A. TEST if it (they) can be reproduced here.
    B. TEST if a bridge must be installed.

Another theme or program could neutralize the one we are currently installing.

18. TEST if there is a harmful program or theme in resonance (echo) or duality (polarity) that could interfere with the new program(s).

Memories of former programs are capable of interfering with the new program.

19. TEST if there are memories attached or linked to former programs that could prevent the integration of this new program in the DNA.
If YES, how many memories are there?

Test each ally with which we will reconnect.

20. TEST if the person can live beyond a state of duality and integrate the reality of having ally/allies ____ within, rather than outside, in his/her genetic code.

21. TEST if the integration of ally/allies ____ within the genetic code creates a destabilization.

22. TEST if the person was communicating with other guides outside himself/herself.
    If YES,
        TEST if there was an alliance.
        If YES,
            TEST if you can put it at zero point or dissolve.

The answer must be NO. If it isn't, this data will be automatically included in the repro-gramming.

23. TEST if this change in ally/allies creates a destabilization at the level of the soul or a distortion at the level of the etheric bodies.

We must get a YES for each ally with whom we are re-establishing a connection.

24. TEST if the person can integrate the reconnection with ally/allies ____ in his/her daily life.

Before installing the program, it may be necessary to input other data.

25. TEST if it is necessary to enter other data in this pro-gram before its installation. If YES, go to Appendix III and follow the instructions to test which data must be entered in this reprogramming. Then, return to the protocol and proceed to the next stage.

2nd Stage – The instal-lation takes into account all the data found in the first stage.

2nd Stage – INSTALLATION OF THE REPROGRAMMING

1. SAY: *I COMMAND that this new program be installed in the nucleus of the master cell of the pineal gland in all lives and all dimensions.*

Insofar as the command is spoken out loud, each item is integrated in the reprogramming. Please use the tone of voice you would use for a prayer or hypnosis as the DNA responds to language spoken in this fashion.

If Point E tests YES , refer to Appendix III and find the area.

2. **SAY: *I COMMAND* that, from the pineal gland, this program reach:**
   A. **the endocrine glands;**
   B. **the brain, the nervous system and the peptides;**
   C. **the cells, the intra and extracellular fluids, the interstitial void, the atoms and the quantum elements (quarks, muons, strands, ...);**
   D. **all of the helixes, chakras, etheric bodies, and the soul;**
   E. **another location** (see Appendix III).

3. **SAY: *I COMMAND* the RNA to support and reconnect itself to this new program.**

The original DNA plan is the underlying pattern that precedes all genetic mutation.

4. **SAY: *I COMMAND* the codons to return to the order of the perfect original program even if there has been an inversion of codes.**

5. **SAY: *I COMMAND* the speed of the photons and the structure of the DNA spiral to adjust themselves.**

6. **SAY: *I COMMAND* that the connection within the corpus callosum of the brain be restored according to the original divine plan.**

The telomere is part of the very structure of the chromosome. It is a protein found at the ends of the chromosomal strands in DNA that protects these strands. In simpler terms, it is the end of each chromosome. The telomerase is an enzyme that acts as the "glue" of the telomere.

7. **SAY: *I COMMAND* the perfect integrity of the telomere and the telomerase.**

Refer to Appendix VII for a list of systems.	**8. SAY: *I COMMAND* that any residues from old programs be eliminated through the appropriate systems.**
	9. SAY: *I COMMAND* that this program be perfectly sealed.
Refer to Appendix I for the definition of Merkabah.	**10. SAY: *I COMMAND* that the Merkabah be perfectly sealed.**
	11. SAY: *I COMMAND* that no radiation affect the DNA or RNA.
	12. SAY: *I COMMAND* that this (these) new ally/allies be reconnected completely, and until further notice, in the brain stem, here and now.
	13. SAY: *I COMMAND* that the reconnection with this (these) ally/allies be perfectly tolerated and integrated and that this occur at zero point.
ESSENTIAL POINT in reprogramming	**14. SAY: *I COMMAND* that the power, the harmony and the purity of this (these) new program be installed in the DNA and be perfectly activated.**

3rd Stage	**3rd Stage – CONCLUSION OF THE PROTOCOL**
The installation of other data may be required before concluding the protocol.	**15. TEST if it is necessary to include other data in the reprogramming for it to be effective, tolerated or integrated.** If YES, go to Appendix III and follow the instructions to test which data must be entered in this reprogramming. Then, return to the protocol and proceed to Step 16.
This closes the protocol.	**16. SAY: *I COMMAND* that this reprogramming be tolerated and integrated, according to the original divine plan, in the frequency of love, even if our helixes have been deactivated in the past.**
This seals the reprogramming.	**17. SAY: *I COMMAND* that this regeneration be complete and sealed, until further notice from ... (the person being reprogrammed).**

PROTOCOL NO. 15

Tolerating the Activation of the 13 Helixes

People who have consciously worked on transforming their DNA by reconnecting and activating the 13 helixes have noted that the process triggers all sorts of changes. For example, some adults grow spiritually while others see the graying process of their hair come to a stop. There are also the less enjoyable symptoms, which generally have a shorter duration but can come back at any time. They could be of a physical nature and may include flu-like symptoms, headaches, occasional nasal congestion with sneezing that seems like hay fever, twenty-four hour flu, hearing problems, earaches, dizziness, digestive problems and more frequent hypoglycemic reactions.

There are also energy symptoms. The individual can sense a vibration throughout the body, especially at bedtime or during relaxation. People can also experience tingling in the arms, hands, legs and feet. The level of hormones can also vary for no apparent reason and some people notice a change in their libido. Several of my students feel more tired or exhausted, with low levels of energy while doing non-strenuous activities and mentioned a desire to sleep longer and more often than usual. Others say they are hyperactive. I notice the quality of dreams is improved, intuition is stronger, and people have a greater ability to gain new understandings about past events.

During the transformation period of my own DNA, I went to bed very early. I experienced huge hormonal changes including several bouts of hypoglycemia and hyperactivity. I also went through moments of tension, anxiety and depression without valid reasons. I was under a lot of stress because I had the impression that something was going on, but I did not know what it was.

It was because of those episodes of flu and inexplicable depression that I was inspired to formulate a protocol whose main objective would be to help us tolerate the change of frequency caused by the reprogramming of our DNA. Since I have installed this new program, there has been a noticeable change in my mood and the inexplicable states of depression no longer have power over me. What a relief!

PROTOCOL NO. 15

Tolerating the Change in Frequency
Due to the Activation of the 13 Helixes

1ˢᵗ Stage of Protocol

1ˢᵗ Stage – PREPARATION

Identifies the object of the protocol as well as the data to be included in the reprogramming process.

Before beginning to test, set your intent by saying: ***I choose to be at zero point even if I don't know how.***

Use kinesiology (or another testing tool) to find the answers. Data thus obtained will be automatically processed by the body's innate intelligence and the genetic code's consciousness, in accordance with your intention.

Refer to Appendix II on how to test a number.

1. **A. TEST the person's percentage of tolerance to frequency changes.**
   B. TEST if the frequency change symptoms are tolerated.

2. **TEST if the person can affirm that it is normal to change frequencies.**

We may obtain a NO for several reasons. We don't need to know why. Simply respect this information.

3. **TEST if you must install the program to tolerate the frequency change in the DNA.**
   If NO,
   A. Do not proceed with this reprogramming.
   B. TEST how much time is needed (days, weeks, months) before testing again.
   If YES,

Finding the exact DNA address is the MAIN PIVOT of all reprogramming. In general, the program is in one gene of a single chromosome.

   A. TEST in which chromosome (1 to 46...) and in which gene (1 to 5,000+) you must install this new program and
   B. TEST how many codons (1 to 30,000+) it comprises.

180

The original DNA plan is the underlying diagram that precedes all genetic mutation. If this information still exists in a latent form, it will automatically be included in the reprogramming.

4. **TEST if the program to tolerate frequency changes already existed in the original divine plan of the person's DNA.**
   If YES,
      A. **TEST if it can be reproduced here.**
      B. **TEST if a bridge must be installed.**

A theme or another program may neutralize the installation of the new program.

5. **TEST if there is a harmful program or theme in resonance (echo) or duality (polarity) that could interfere with the new program.**

Memories of former programs are capable of interfering with the new program.

6. **TEST if there are memories attached or linked to former programs that could prevent the integration of this new program in the DNA.**
   If YES, how many memories are there?

7. **TEST at which percentage the person is able to let himself/ herself go in the frequency change process.**

The answer must be NO. If it isn't, this data will be automatically included in the reprogramming.

8. **TEST if there is an allergy to frequency change in the form of:**
   A. **auto-immunity towards the old frequency;**
   B. **auto-immunity towards the new frequency.**

Test each word.

9. **TEST if there is a genetic rivalry because of the frequency change,**
   A. **at the biochemical level: carbon, hydrogen, oxygen, nitrogen, other;**
   B. **at the electromagnetic level: speed (too fast or slow) and frequency (too high or low) of the electrons;**
   C. **at the extracellular or intracellular level;**
      if YES,
         TEST the percentage of integrity (intra or extracellular);

D. at the hormonal and the peptides level;

E. at the level of the systems: nervous, gastro-intestinal and psycho-neuro-immunological;

F. at the cellular and atomic level: cells, atoms, quantum elements (quarks, muons, strands, ...);

G. **other** (see Appendix III).

Test each word.

10. TEST if the metabolic waste coming from the change of frequency is being completely eliminated.
If NO,
TEST which system(s) is (are) at cause:
A. lymphatic
B. hepatic
C. digestive or intestinal
D. renal
E. respiratory
F. nervous
G. **other** (see Appendix VII).

Test each word.

11. TEST if the mitochondria and the chromosomes are in rivalry for the same material (bases or amino acids) or if there is another rivalry in the nucleus of the cell, on the energetic level, because of the change of frequency.

We must obtain a NO for Steps 12 to 14. If the opposite occurs, the data will be automatically included in the reprogramming by the innate intelligence.

12. TEST if there are antibodies against the new frequency.

13. TEST if the frequency change creates a distortion at the level of the aura.

14. TEST if the etheric bodies are out of sync because of the frequency change.

15. TEST if the activation of the parts of the brain that were previously inactive is tolerated.

16. TEST if the electromagnetic fields of the 13 helixes cause a nervous disorder of an electric nature.

17. TEST if the crystalline structure of the helixes is activated by the hypothalamus, and if yes, TEST at which percentage.

18. TEST if radiation affects the wave frequency of the 13 helixes.

19. TEST if miasmas or transgenerational memories are interfering with the frequency change.

Test each word as the person speaks them aloud.

20. TEST if the person knows that he/she can change frequencies and still be loved.

21. TEST if the person's intuition and energy are amplified proportionally to the frequency change.

The percentage tested will be automatically included in the reprogramming.

22. A. TEST if the magnetic field needs to be ionized.
    B. TEST the percentage of integrity of the negative and positive ions.

It must be 100%. The blood-brain barrier is a sanguine filter which only allows tiny molecules such as glucose to pass through the brain.

23. TEST the percentage of integrity of the blood-brain barrier.

Refer to Appendix II on how to test a number.

24. TEST if it is necessary to repair one or several gene(s) in a chromosome.
    If YES, go to Protocol 8 and proceed with the repair(s) before moving to the next step.

Refer to Appendix II on how to test a number.

25. TEST if there exists a familial pattern that interferes with, or blocks, the frequency change.
    If YES,
         A. TEST how many generations it goes back.
         B. TEST if it must be put at zero point or dissolved.

Before installing the program, it may be necessary to input other data.

26. **TEST if it is necessary to enter other data in this program before its installation.** If YES, go to Appendix III and follow the instructions to test which data must be entered in this reprogramming. Then, return to the protocol and proceed to the next stage.

2nd Stage – The installation takes into account all the data found in the first stage.

2nd Stage – INSTALLATION OF THE REPROGRAMMING

Insofar as the command is spoken out loud, each item is integrated in the reprogramming. Please use the tone of voice you would use for a prayer or hypnosis as the DNA responds to language spoken in this fashion.

1. **SAY:** *I COMMAND that this new program be installed in the nucleus of the master cell of the pineal gland in all lives and all dimensions.*

2. **SAY:** *I COMMAND that, from the pineal gland, this program reach:*
   A. *the endocrine glands;*
   B. *the brain, the nervous system and the peptides;*
   C. *the cells, the intra and extracellular fluids, the interstitial void, the atoms and the quantum elements (quarks, muons, strands, ...);*
   D. *all of the helixes, chakras, etheric bodies, and the soul;*
   E. *another location* (see Appendix III).

If Point E tests YES, refer to Appendix III and find the area.

3. **SAY:** *I COMMAND the RNA to support and reconnect itself to this new program.*

The original DNA plan is the underlying pattern that precedes all genetic mutation.

4. **SAY:** *I COMMAND the codons to return to the order of the perfect original program even if there has been an inversion of codes.*

5. **SAY:** *I COMMAND the speed of the photons and the structure of the DNA spiral to adjust themselves.*

6. **SAY:** *I COMMAND that the connection within the corpus callosum of the brain be restored according to the original divine plan.*

The telomere is part of the very structure of the chromosome. It is a protein found at the ends of the chromosomal strands in DNA that protects these strands. In simpler terms, it is the end of each chromosome. The telomerase is an enzyme that acts as the "glue" of the telomere.

7. SAY: *I COMMAND* the perfect integrity of the telomere and the telomerase.

Refer to Appendix VII for a list of systems.

8. SAY: *I COMMAND* that any residues from old programs be eliminated through the appropriate systems.

9. SAY: *I COMMAND* that this program be perfectly sealed.

Refer to Appendix I for the definition of Merkabah.

10. SAY: *I COMMAND* that the Merkabah be perfectly sealed.

11. SAY: *I COMMAND* that no radiation affect the DNA or RNA.

12. SAY: *I COMMAND* that this (these) new program(s) be installed completely, and until further notice, in the brain stem, here and now.

13. SAY: *I COMMAND* that the reconnection of this new program be perfectly tolerated and integrated and that this occurs at zero point.

ESSENTIAL POINT in reprogramming

14. SAY: *I COMMAND* that the power, the harmony and the purity of this (these) new programs be installed in the DNA and be perfectly activated.

3rd Stage **3rd Stage – CONCLUSION OF THE PROTOCOL**

The installation of other data may be required before concluding the protocol.

15. TEST if it is necessary to include other data in the reprogramming for it to be effective, tolerated or integrated. If YES, go to Appendix III and follow the instructions to test which data must be entered in this reprogramming. Then, return to the protocol and proceed to Step 16.

This closes the protocol.

16. SAY: *I COMMAND that this reprogramming be tolerated and integrated, according to the original divine plan, in the frequency of love, even if our helixes have been deactivated in the past.*

This seals the reprogramming.

17. SAY: *I COMMAND that this regeneration be complete and sealed, until further notice from ... (the person being reprogrammed).*

Line S. wrote the following regarding this protocol.

For the past ten years, I have been working as a chartered accountant in companies. My leadership skills have enabled me to develop great relationships. Reprogramming my DNA using kinesiology has been a great tool in helping me to develop extraordinary contact with other human beings.

During the reprogramming process, I lost eight kilograms and my self-esteem improved tremendously. DNA has become a powerful tool in my life regarding change. I currently find it easier to deal with what I want to see happen on a physical, emotional, spiritual or mental level. With experience, I have a better understanding of the protocols and how carefully they have been designed. They are efficient and my body tolerates them very well. I also appreciate the fact that they are accessible. All I needed to do was understand the basics and become aware that, if I use the energy of intention, I can change almost anything. Now that I have this tool, I know that I can improve my life without having to sail the seas of pain.

PROTOCOL NO. 16

Being Perfectly Sealed

I have noticed that many of my clients are hypersensitive and this was at the root of their problems. Some allow the emotions of their loved ones or of the people they work with to invade them. Others are easily affected by the full moon. Some people react badly in crowds, or to the electromagnetic pollution of shopping centers, or to signals emitted by computers, telecommunications or satellites.

Obviously these people have great difficulties establishing clear limits. Visualizing protective screens or trying to stay in a happy disposition did not seem to be enough. Even white light protection techniques were of no help. I had also noticed that, in general, these people were of a sensitive nature and often more intuitive than most. I got the idea to develop a protocol just for them, designed to seal their DNA. If we are 100% sealed we will be able to manifest our desires more easily because there will be no more interference.

Multidimensionality

Before you begin the work on this protocol, I would like to clarify the term "multidimensionality" included in Step 17. We refer to "multidimensionality" when discussing the 13 helixes of DNA. When our DNA will be completely re-connected and harmonized, we will access our "multidimensionality". This term, however, has never been clearly defined. To understand its true meaning, I relied on concepts in quantum physics in which time is non-linear.

Imagine that our parental soul is a big sun and that each ray represents an incarnation (present, past or future). When we are in the center of this big sun, we have access to more than one life, to more than one time-space continuum at a particular moment. To remain stable, we must concentrate on one of the rays that represents our current incarnation. However, the distance between the rays may not always be precise or set and these timelines may even touch or intertwine.

Seen from this perspective, "multidimensionality" could be the source of some of the discomfort felt by a hypersensitive person. In fact, it is possible that these people have the ability, although unconscious and non-mastered, to live or to be in several dimensions at the same time, placing them temporarily into a state of confusion and instability.

Whether or not this is "multidimensionality", if you recognize any one of the states of vulnerability that I mentioned, I suggest that you use the Protocol 16 to seal your DNA without having to build an impenetrable wall to isolate yourself. From now on, you can decide when you want to remain sensitive to others and to your environment.

PROTOCOL NO. 16

Being Perfectly Sealed

1st Stage of Protocol

1st Stage – PREPARATION

Identifies the object of the protocol as well as the data to be included in the reprogramming process.

Before beginning to test, set your intent by saying: ***I choose to be at zero point even if I don't know how***.

Use kinesiology (or another testing tool) to find the answers. Data thus obtained will be automatically processed by the body's innate intelligence and the genetic code's consciousness, in accordance with your intention.

We may obtain a NO for several reasons. We don't need to know why. Simply respect this information.

1. **A. TEST if you must install a program in the DNA to be 100% sealed.**
    A. in general, OR
    B. in regard to a particular situation to be included in this session.
    If YES,
    > **TEST which specific situation.**

We may obtain a NO for several reasons. We don't need to know why. Simply respect this information.

  B. TEST if it is appropriate to install this program now.
    If NO,
    A. Do not proceed with this reprogramming.
    B. TEST how much time is needed (days, weeks, months) before testing again.
    If YES

Finding the exact DNA address is the MAIN PIVOT of all reprogramming. In general, the program is in one gene of a single chromosome.

    A. TEST in which chromosome (1 to 46...) **and in which gene** (1 to 5,000+) **you must install this new program and**
    B. TEST how many codons (1 to 30,000+) **it comprises.**

189

The original DNA plan is the underlying diagram that precedes all genetic mutation. If this information still exists in a latent form, it will automatically be included in the reprogramming.

2. **TEST if the program to be 100% sealed already existed in the original divine plan of the person's DNA.**
   If YES,
   A. **TEST if it can be reproduced here.**
   B. **TEST if a bridge must be installed.**

A theme or another program may neutralize the installation of the new program.

3. **TEST if there is a harmful program or theme in resonance (echo) or duality (polarity) that could interfere with the new program.**

Memories of former programs are capable of interfering with the new program.

4. **TEST if there are memories attached or linked to former programs that could prevent the integration of this new program in the DNA.**
   If YES, how many memories are there?

We must obtain a YES. If we test another percentage, the data will be automatically included in the reprogramming.

5. **TEST if the person has access to the program to be "100% sealed."**

We must get 100%.

6. **TEST which percentage of the cells remember what it is to be 100% sealed.**

Test each word. If we get a NO for Points C, D and E, verify which etheric body(ies), chakra(s) or helix(es) does not test.

Go to Appendix III to find which other location needs to be sealed at 100%.

7. **TEST if the following elements can be 100% sealed:**
   A. **the soul;**
   B. **the Merkabah;**
   C. **all of the etheric bodies;**
   D. **all of the chakras;**
   E. **the 13 helixes;**
   F. **the physical body;**
   G. **the person's home, workplace, his/her car, etc.;**
   H. **other** (see Appendix III).

8. **TEST if there is a blockage preventing the person from being 100% sealed.**

We must get a YES.

9. **TEST if the person can live while being "100% sealed."**

We must get a NO.

10. **TEST if the person still needs to not be "100% sealed."**

The answer must be NO. If it isn't, this data will be automatically included in the reprogramming.

11. **TEST if the person is attached to not being "100% sealed."**

12. **TEST if the program to be 100% sealed is perfectly anchored in daily life.**

The answer must be YES. If it isn't, this data will be automatically included in the reprogramming.

13. **A. TEST if the person can perceive the difference in his/her body between being completely sealed and partially sealed.**

To be tired for no reason, to fall into self criticism, or to feel unaligned, are all references indicating that one is not 100% sealed.

B. TEST if the person's genetic code contains the program permitting him/her to feel in his/her physical body whether he/she is "100% sealed."

C. TEST if the person's genetic code contains the program permitting him/her to feel whether his/her environment is "100% sealed."

D. TEST if the person knows how to recognize his/her referential mode, a system of signals that alerts him/her to the fact that he/she (or his/her environment) is not 100% sealed.

Refer to Appendix II to know how to test.

E. TEST if you can activate or reactivate the programs so that the person can feel in his/her physical body if he/she is "100% sealed" and if his/her environment is "100% sealed."

F. TEST if you can include in the new program a code permitting the person to completely seal himself/herself and his/her environment automatically when he/she perceives that it is not sealed anymore.

Test every word.

14. **TEST if the person can integrate being "100% sealed" at the level of:**
   A. the endocrine glands;
   B. the brain, the nervous system and the peptides;

C. the five senses;

D. the 13 helixes, the chakras, the etheric bodies and the soul;

E. another location (see Appendix III).

15. TEST if the person can manifest all of his/her desires while remaining "100% sealed."

Test each word.

16. TEST if the person is able:

A. to stay open to the universe, even if he/she is "100% sealed";

B. to be in contact with other dimensions, even if he/she is "100% sealed";

C. to be in contact with others, even if he/she is "100% sealed";

D. to be inspired, even if he/she is "100% sealed";

E. to be himself/herself, even if he/she is "100% sealed";

F. to know who he/she is, even if he/she is "100% sealed";

G. to be psychically whole, even if he/she is "100% sealed";

H. other intent (see Appendix V) **even if he/she is "100% sealed."**

Test each word.

17. TEST if there are miasmas, karmic implants, or trans-generational memories, past wounds or future anticipations to be put at zero point, or dissolved.

18. A. TEST if the density of the etheric bodies is weighed down when the person is not "100% sealed."

B. TEST if the person's genetic code contains the program permitting him/her to reduce the density of the etheric bodies when he/she becomes sealed.

19. TEST if the person can stay connected to his/her 13 helixes while remaining "100% sealed."

Before installing the program, it may be necessary to input other data.

20. TEST if it is necessary to enter other data in this program before its installation. If YES, go to Appendix III and follow the instructions to test which data must be entered in this reprogramming. Then, return to the protocol and proceed to the next stage.

2nd Stage – The installation takes into account all the data found in the first stage.

2nd Stage – INSTALLATION OF THE REPROGRAMMING

Insofar as the command is spoken out loud, each item is integrated in the reprogramming. Please use the tone of voice you would use for a prayer or hypnosis as the DNA responds to language spoken in this fashion.

1. **SAY: *I COMMAND* that this new program be installed in the nucleus of the master cell of the pineal gland in all lives and all dimensions.**

2. **SAY: *I COMMAND* that, from the pineal gland, this program reach:**
   A. **the endocrine glands;**
   B. **the brain, the nervous system and the peptides;**
   C. **the cells, the intra and extracellular fluids, the interstitial void, the atoms and the quantum elements (quarks, muons, strands, ...);**
   D. **all of the helixes, chakras, etheric bodies, and the soul;**

If Point E tests YES, refer to Appendix III and find the area.

   E. **another location** (see Appendix III).

3. **SAY: *I COMMAND* the RNA to support and reconnect itself to this new program.**

The original DNA plan is the underlying pattern that precedes all genetic mutation.

4. **SAY: *I COMMAND* the codons to return to the order of the perfect original program even if there has been an inversion of codes.**

5. **SAY: *I COMMAND* the speed of the photons and the structure of the DNA spiral to adjust themselves.**

6. **SAY: *I COMMAND* that the connection within the corpus callosum of the brain be restored according to the original divine plan.**

The telomere is part of the very structure of the chromosome. It is a protein found at the ends of the chromosomal strands in DNA that protects these strands. In simpler terms, it is the end of each chromosome. The telomerase is an enzyme that acts as the "glue" of the telomere.

7. **SAY: *I COMMAND* the perfect integrity of the telomere and the telomerase.**

Refer to Appendix VII for a list of systems.

8. **SAY: *I COMMAND* that any residues from old programs be eliminated through the appropriate systems.**

9. **SAY: *I COMMAND* that this program be perfectly sealed.**

Refer to Appendix I for the definition of Merkabah.

10. **SAY: *I COMMAND* that the Merkabah be perfectly sealed.**

11. **SAY: *I COMMAND* that no radiation affect the DNA or RNA.**

12. **SAY: *I COMMAND* that this (these) new program(s) be installed completely, and until further notice, in the brain stem, here and now.**

13. **SAY: *I COMMAND* that the reconnection of this (these) new program(s) be perfectly tolerated and integrated and that this occurs at zero point.**

ESSENTIAL POINT in reprogramming

14. **SAY: *I COMMAND* that the power, the harmony and the purity of this new program be installed in the DNA and be perfectly activated.**

3rd Stage

3rd Stage – CONCLUSION OF THE PROTOCOL

The installation of other data may be required before concluding the protocol.

15. **TEST if it is necessary to include other data in the reprogramming for it to be effective, tolerated or integrated.** If YES, go to Appendix III and follow the instructions to test which data must be entered in this reprogramming. Then, return to the protocol and proceed to Step 16.

This closes the protocol.

16. **SAY: *I COMMAND* that this reprogramming be tolerated and integrated, according to the original divine plan, in the frequency of love, even if our helixes have been deactivated in the past.**

This seals the reprogramming.

17. **SAY: *I COMMAND* that this regeneration be complete and sealed, until further notice from ... (the person being reprogrammed).**

Micheline N. wrote the following regarding this protocol:

I was not feeling very well. It was as if the inside of my head contained a vibrating mass that kept me in a kind of trance. I felt unstable and nothing seemed to be circulating properly. One treatment was enough to correct different points in my body and to reprogram new data. I was only 10% sealed. As soon as Bruno started the protocol, I felt like pieces were breaking away from the mass inside my head and settling themselves all around my skull like water bubbles rising up to the surface. Everything then settled, the tension left, and I had a peaceful, easy feeling. I then calmly got behind the wheel of my car and was able to drive away.

PROTOCOL NO. 17

DNA and the Spiritual Quest

The more I delved into my work on DNA, the easier it was for me to go within myself. I can now close my eyes and rest inside the spirals of my 13 helixes. As well, after developing these protocols on a variety of subjects falling under almost every aspect of human life, it seemed logical to use this reprogramming power to guide me in my spiritual quest. The result was Protocol 17.

After installing this protocol on myself, I spent two days in a state of absolute bliss. I was no longer alone, lost in the universe; instead I felt united with the Source. This brought about an implosion within me that finally enabled me to meditate without continuously fighting against discomfort and a wandering mind. Since this experience, I have felt more connected and time does not appear to drag on. So here is the protocol … wishing you successful meditation!

PROTOCOL NO. 17

Implosion Within Our DNA

1ˢᵗ Stage of Protocol

1ˢᵗ Stage – PREPARATION

Identifies the object of the protocol as well as the data to be included in the reprogramming process.

Before beginning to test, set your intent by saying: ***I choose to be at zero point even if I don't know how.***

Use kinesiology (or another testing tool) to find the answers. Data thus obtained will be automatically processed by the body's innate intelligence and the genetic code's conscious-ness, in accordance with your intention.

Refer to the main text and Appendix I for the definition on "implo-sion."

1. **TEST if the person is able to create an implosion within his/ her own genetic code at the new zero point frequency.**
   A. in general, OR
   B. in regard to a particular situation to be included in this session.
      If YES,
         TEST which specific situation.

We may obtain a NO for several reasons. We don't need to know why. Simply respect this information.

Refer to Appendix II on how to test a number.

Finding the exact DNA address is the MAIN PIVOT of all reprogramming. In general, the program is in one gene of a single chromosome.

2. **TEST if you can install a program so that the person is able to create an implosion within his/her own genetic code.**
   If NO,
      A. DO NOT proceed with the reconnection now.
      B. TEST how much time is needed (days, weeks, months) before testing once more to reconnect.
   If YES,
      A. TEST in which chromosome (1 to 46...) **and in which gene** (1 to 5,000+) **you must install this new program and**
      B. TEST how many codons (1 to 30,000+) **it comprises.**

196

The original DNA plan is the underlying diagram that precedes all genetic mutation. If this information still exists in a latent form, it will automatically be included in the repro-gramming.

3. **TEST if the program to create an implosion within one's DNA already existed in the original divine plan of the person's DNA.**
   If YES,
   A. **TEST if it can be reproduced here.**
   B. **TEST if a bridge must be installed.**

A theme or another program may neutral-ize the installation of the new program.

4. **TEST if there is a harmful program or theme in resonance (echo) or duality (polarity) that could interfere with the new program.**

Memories of former programs are capable of interfering with the new program.

5 **TEST if there are memories attached or linked to former programs that could prevent the integration in the DNA of this new program.**
   If YES, how many memories are there?

6. **TEST you must install a bridge between the hypothala-mus and the frontal lobe.**

Refer to Appendix II on how to test a number.

There could be hun-dreds, maybe thou-sands, of fragments.

7. A. **TEST how many fragments have separated them-selves from the person because of this type of event OR what percentage of the person is fragmented and separated because of this implosion.**
   B. **TEST if it is appropriate to bring these fragments into the present at zero point and to anchor them in the DNA.**

8. **TEST if an alliance blocks the implosion.**

9. **TEST if the soul is in a state of shock and if this pre-vents the implosion.**

Test each word.

10. **TEST if the ego is at risk of fragmenting or being desta-bilized by the implosion at zero point.**

Test each word.

11. TEST if the implosion could destabilize or fragment:
   A. the endocrine glands;
   B. the brain, the nervous system and the peptides;
   C. the cells, the intra and extracellular fluids, the interstitial void, the atoms and the quantum elements (quarks, muons, strands,...);
   D. all of the helixes, chakras, etheric bodies and the soul;
   E. another location (see Appendix III).

12. TEST if it is necessary to adjust the helixes' electromagnetic field to facilitate the implosion.

13. TEST if it is necessary to install a new quantum particle in the atom to allow the implosion.

The answer must be YES. If it isn't, this data will be automatically included in the reprogramming.

14. TEST if the implosion is 100% tolerated.

We speak here of benefits such as abundance, security, health, etc.

15. TEST if the person is able to live with the success of the implosion.

16. TEST if the person can transmit the benefits of this implosion to his/her physical body and to his/her earthly reality.
   If NO,
      TEST if a bridge must be installed.

17. TEST if the person is able to "multidimensionally" reconnect to himself/herself thanks to the implosion.

18. TEST if the person is able to return to the original state of Unity thanks to the implosion in his/her genetic code.

Before installing the program, it may be necessary to input other data.

19. TEST if it is necessary to enter other data in this program before its installation. If YES, go to Appendix III and follow the instructions to test which data must be entered in this reprogramming. Then, return to the protocol and proceed to the next stage.

2nd Stage – The installation takes into account all the data found in the first Stage.

2nd Stage – INSTALLATION OF THE REPROGRAMMING

1. **SAY: I COMMAND that this new program be installed in the nucleus of the master cell of the pineal gland in all lives and all dimensions.**

Insofar as the command is spoken out loud, each item is integrated in the reprogramming. Please use the tone of voice you would use for a prayer or hypnosis as the DNA responds to language spoken in this fashion.

If Point E tests YES , refer to Appendix III and find the area.

2. **SAY: I COMMAND that, from the pineal gland, this program reach:**
   A. the endocrine glands;
   B. the brain, the nervous system and the peptides;
   C. the cells, the intra and extracellular fluids, the interstitial void, the atoms and the quantum elements (quarks, muons, strands, ...);
   D. all of the helixes, chakras, etheric bodies, and the soul;
   E. another location (see Appendix III).

3. **SAY: I COMMAND the RNA to support and reconnect itself to this new program.**

The original DNA plan is the underlying pattern that precedes all genetic mutation.

4. **SAY: I COMMAND the codons to return to the order of the perfect original program even if there has been an inversion of codes.**

5. **SAY: I COMMAND the speed of the photons and the structure of the DNA spiral to adjust themselves.**

6. **SAY: I COMMAND that the connection within the corpus callosum of the brain be restored according to the original divine plan.**

The telomere is part of the very structure of the chromosome. It is a protein found at the ends of the chromosomal strands in DNA that protects these strands. In simpler terms, it is the end of each chromosome. The telomerase is an enzyme that acts as the "glue" of the telomere.

7. **SAY: I COMMAND the perfect integrity of the telomere and the telomerase.**

Refer to Appendix VII for a list of systems.

8. SAY: *I COMMAND that any residues from old programs be eliminated through the appropriate systems.*

9. SAY: *I COMMAND that this program be perfectly sealed.*

Refer to Appendix I for the definition of Merkabah.

10. SAY: *I COMMAND that the Merkabah be perfectly sealed.*

11. SAY: *I COMMAND that no radiation affect the DNA or RNA.*

12. SAY: *I COMMAND that this new program be installed completely, and until further notice, in the brain stem, here and now.*

13. SAY: *I COMMAND that the reconnection of this new program be perfectly tolerated and integrated and that this occurs at zero point.*

ESSENTIAL POINT in reprogramming

14. SAY: *I COMMAND that the power, the harmony and the purity of this (these) new programs be installed in the DNA and be perfectly activated.*

3rd Stage

3rd Stage – CONCLUSION OF THE PROTOCOL

The installation of other data may be required before concluding the protocol.

15. **TEST if it is necessary to include other data in the reprogramming for it to be effective, tolerated or integrated.** If YES, go to Appendix III and follow the instructions to test which data must be entered in this reprogramming. Then, return to the protocol and proceed to Step 16.

This closes the protocol.

16. SAY: *I COMMAND that this reprogramming be tolerated and integrated, according to the original divine plan, in the frequency of love, even if our helixes have been deactivated in the past.*

This seals the reprogramming.

17. SAY: *I COMMAND that this regeneration be complete and sealed, until further notice from ... (the person being reprogrammed).*

Access to New Scenarios

Now that you have reached the end of the book, you know how to formulate programs so that they present unlimited possibilities. By understanding genetic engineering protocols, we can now create the reality we want. We are the masters of our behaviours and programs.

We are the experts of the third dimension. We are responsible for saying what we want, how we feel, what makes us uncomfortable, and what makes us happy. This new way of thinking, the creation of new realities, the state of love, the lack of interference regarding our DNA, and the activation of the 13 allies within us, all point toward one conclusion: our sovereignty over our own DNA. I live among people who perfectly understand the way life works on Earth. These people have taken it upon themselves to restructure and redefine the human genome. The genome revolution is not only taking place in the laboratory. It is globally initiated on Earth by those who are again co-creators of their own DNA through the power of intention.

One of the most difficult issues to resolve will be to find an adequate balance between our reprogramming vision and trusting in our own ability to recode with no other authority except our own. Let's experiment with the protocols and enjoy the changes in our relationships, our health and our surroundings. And since scientists particularly ignore the function of approximately 97% of DNA, let us be the ones to redefine it!

You can imagine that, as a rebel and innovator, I have devoted myself to opening, introducing and firmly rooting the frequency of love in the third dimension. This was the driving force behind the creation of the reprogramming protocols that I presented throughout this book.

Conclusion

After activating our genetic code, we will feel more intuitive, not as powerless, and not as limited by never-ending processes. Some people report feeling younger and in better health. Our DNA is not static—therein lies the greatest discovery of this century. By changing our way of being, we will create a new race or return to the original race.

One day, in Arizona, I met a therapist who worked on DNA. She was the one who gave me the idea for the chart of 13 helixes. She did not work with kinesiology, but she asked questions as ludicrous as my own, if not more so, and the answers came to her through prayer and intention. When I visited her, she told me that she was really happy to meet me, since she rarely had the opportunity to get to know another person whose helixes had been reconnected and who was aware of it. She seemed to receive her information through channelling, but, as I mentioned, I only communicate with my good old innate intelligence! She told me that I was initiated into the third level of Melchisedech and that I could remotely heal someone in the astral world while I slept at night! She asked me whether I knew that and I answered that I had no idea. Without realizing it, I had arrived where I am today, simply by reprogramming my DNA and becoming able to recognize my multidimensional self so that it could merge with my life mission. DNA is very powerful once it is reconnected!

At this point in time, I had already been practicing Tantra for a few years. I had varying levels of success until I integrated my 13 helixes. After that, I was able to reach the spiritual levels attained by the initiated, as described in sacred texts. I could easily travel with my spouse into the circular universe of the cosmic orbit without any restriction, between the 12th helix that links us to the Source and the 13th helix that firmly roots us in darkness.

Our ultimate goal is not only to reactivate all our helixes but to live in a circular perspective. It is like we were in the center of a pie and each situation was being perceived as one of thirteen portions instead of the usual two. This circular vision brings compassion, understanding, abundance, humility and self-love.

When people tell me that I have a good life, great children and that I look good, I always say that it is my DNA and my intention that have brought all that to me. It may appear that, compared to other people, everything is easy for me. However, I have four children and a dog, and still have to do the dishes. I experience the dangers of winter snowstorms. I feel cold in the winter and hot in the summer. I can burst out laughing or cry for no reason. In fact, I do not have any definite proof that the DNA programs are infallible although certain people exhibit some results (no more gray hair, never sick, etc.). I myself have much more vitality and I no longer become depressed. In my opinion the real proof lies in the harmony and the ease we have in talking about "real things" and the wonderful synchronicity which happens in our lives.

From the time I was very young, I knew instinctively that reality as it appears is not the only option. I am the youngest of seven children, and I was born under the sign of Aries with the number nine as my numerological path. I came to this planet to experiment new beginnings and see old cycles end.

Now that my 13 helixes are reconnected, and from what I have discovered on the path up to now, I can finally say that I am GOD/GODDESS. I trust it will be the same for you.

Lexicon

Chromosome: A chromosome is a combination of a variable number of genes. Current studies show that a single chromosome could contain more than 5,000 genes. Human DNA contains 46 chromosomes or "chromosomal strands."

Codon: Codons are the building blocks of the gene (see Gene). The basic components of DNA are four nucleic acids: adenine (A), thymine (T), guanine (G) and cytosine (C). These four nucleic acids combine into specific pairs: AT or TA, GC or CG. These pairs then join three by three to form what we call a codon. The "phrase" "AT CG GC" is an example of a codon.
There are 64 different ways of combining the pairs of nucleic acids to form codons, which is the same as saying there are 64 possible types of codons. Only 20 active combinations out of the 64 possible ones are found in humans worldwide, in addition to three other combinations considered to be code "triggers" or "interrupters". This means that 41 out of the 64 possible codon forms are not activated.
A gene (genetic program or code) may be made up of only two codons or a very large number of codons. For example, a team of specialists from Toronto Hospital discovered a gene (probably the one that controls the brain's structure) that may have 100,000 or more codons.

Fragments: Every time we experience a lot of stress or dissociation, we run the risk of having a psychic accident through which we lose part of our being (or self). Spiritual texts refer to this type of accident as "self-fragmentation." According to some authors, these fragmented parts of our being could have their own life while others have even suggested that this fragmentation is one of the causes of the Earth's overpopulation.
Whatever the reason for fragmentation, it is clear that the more we connect our lost helixes, the more we can take back ownership of these fragments of our

being, which are no longer taking part in our conscious personal reality.

According to some sources that I found on the Internet, gathering together all our fragments would be one way of accessing higher levels of consciousness. Moreover, I noticed that one of the most powerful and best ways of accelerating our evolution with ease and joy is to include all our fragments when formulating our intentions and then they also benefit from our reprogramming.

Gene: A gene is a component of a chromosome (see Chromosome). Made up of a series of codons (See Codon), it is a "code" or "program" that shapes and determines how a hereditary characteristic will appear. According to scientists, the human genome contains between 90,000 and 100,000 genes, that is an approximate average of 5,000 genes per chromosome, but some chromosomes may contain far fewer and others far more.

Hologram: Holograms or holographic insertions are a "false" or "virtual" reality, which can be mistaken for concrete three-dimensional reality. Holograms are events that are created, produced and inserted vibrationally into our life to give us the illusion that they are part of our reality. However, holographic insertions are energy fields that are different from that of reality. They vibrate at an incredible speed, which enables them to be detected through kinesiology or any other intuitive method. When faced with a hologram, a sensitive person will have the feeling that something is not right or a bit strange. Something strikes them as "off", even though it is difficult to discern what. This is due to the vibratory helixes of DNA that are not reacting correctly in the presence of these holograms.

Merkabah: There are three fields superposed on one another around our body: physical, mental and emotional. If these fields are turned by connecting the mental, the emotional and the physical body, then the mental field turns towards the left, the emotional towards the right and the physical remains immobile. When these fields turn at a very precise speed and in a specific way, it may create a sphere.

Miasmas: A miasma is a deficiency, an emptiness, or an energy weakness that makes us more vulnerable to certain pathologies or a psychological imbalance. Although miasmas are vibrational, they can manifest physically in the cells and molecules if certain conditions are triggered. These manifestations of energy can affect us mildly through slight weaknesses or seriously through serious mutations or changes.

To establish a link, there must be temporary energetic compatibility between an individual and the miasma's environment. This could result from a shock (good or bad), for example. Such a shock could open a door to the miasma, which then settles itself as a smaller disjointed reality. The body reacts to this intrusion by creating an energy buffer around the miasmas to protect itself from the intruder. A miasma can thus stay entrapped both in terms of energy and molecularly for a long time. As long, in fact, as there is no trigger. It does not bother the person other than when the vital energy is no longer available to maintain this protective wall. The miasma then becomes part of a person's molecular structure and a person can then genetically pass on this **junk or random DNA** to future generations. The energy of a miasma, freed by a trigger, can then end up causing health problems. In fact, the main cause of certain allergies could have nothing to do with the environment or the immune system, but rather they could be triggered by the activity of a once dormant miasma. The only way to eliminate the allergies is by treating the miasma itself.

Telomerase: The telomerase is an enzyme that acts as the "glue" of the telomere (see Telomere).

Telomere: The telomere is part of the very structure of the chromosome. It is a protein found at the ends of the chromosomal strands in DNA that protects these strands. In simpler terms, it is the end of each chromosome.

When a telomere deteriorates, the cell dies, whereas when a telomere is healthy, it allows normal cells to live longer. During cell division, the telomere may become lost or damaged. This may result in abnormalities in cellular multiplication or may completely interrupt cell division. If the telomere is affected, we lose genetic material. This degeneration of genetic material is responsible for aging and disease.

Appendix II

Kinesiology

Two Techniques for Finger-Testing Kinesiology

The word **kinesiology** is derived from the Greek language and means the "study of movement." Traditional kinesiology studies muscle movements and muscular resistance in relation to the internal dynamics of the body.

The kinesiology test used in reprogramming kinesiology is a muscular resistance test that allows us to interpret the response of the body. This is why we can say that with reprogramming kinesiology, we practice a truly democratic therapy because it is not the therapist, in a dominating position, who decides what needs to be done anymore. Rather, it is the innate intelligence of the body itself, thanks to a system of questions and answers, that dictates the progression to follow.

In a kinesiology test, the object is not to measure strength, but to observe changes in muscle resistance. In the classis sugar test, the therapist first measures the natural resistance of the arm muscles by applying pressure downwards, then puts a sugar packet on the subject and tests the muscular resistance again in the same arm. If the sugar has a negative effect on the individual (which happens nine times out of ten), resistance is definitely lower and the arm lowers (or falls) when subjected to the same downward pressure. If the sugar does not affect the individual, resistance remains intact. This is not a question of fatigue. If the test is performed again after removing the sugar, resistance becomes normal again.

There is more than one method of kinesiology testing and we introduce two in this appendix. We recommend that you use the first method, because it is the most practical, since it only uses one hand. It is possible, however, that you may need to practice it for a while before obtaining valid answers.

Basic Principle

Whatever the chosen methor, the basic principle stays the same:

1. You ask a question leading to a "yes" or "no" answer and you measure the resistance.

2. If resistance decreases, it means YES. If resistance remains stable or increases, it means NO.

Here are both methods. Then, in the next section, we will learn how to find answers to questions which include numbers.

Method 1 – The Two Fingers

In this method, to test muscular resistance, you place the middle finger on the index, with both fingers held straight. The middle finger exerts a downwards pressure, as if to bend the index at the base joint, while the index resists.

1. Ask a question.
2. Exert a pressure on the index finger using the middle finger.
3. If the index bends (which is generally felt at the level of the joint nearest to the palm), it means YES. If, on the contrary, it has resisted without bending, it means NO.

If you have difficulty obtaining consistent answers, you may need to "teach" (say, out loud, to …) your fingers that a slack signifies a YES and that, inversely, the upkeep of tension (or the increase thereof) will be understood as a NO.

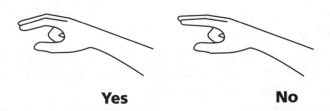

Yes   **No**

Method 2 – The Circuit

In this method, you form a circuit by firmly connecting the thumb and the pinky of one hand. The test will consist of attempting to break the circuit by exerting a pressure with the index and the thumb of the other hand, inserted in the circle formed by the circuit. If the circuit is broken (therefore the resistance has diminished), that means YES. If, on the contrary, the circuit remains closed (the resistance was maintained), then it means NO.

The Fingers of the Circuit

A. <u>For right-handed people:</u>
Raise the left hand and join the end of the left thumb with the end of the left auricular.

B. <u>For left-handed people:</u>
Raise the right hand and join the end of the right thumb with the end of the right auricular.

You have thus formed a circuit.

It is important to maintain an equal and continuous pressure between the fingers of the circuit, when you test. It is necessary to put just enough strength for the fingers to feel alive and connected, and to let the fingers decide if they will resist or slacken.

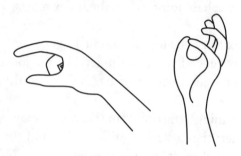

The Testing Fingers

To test the circuit, join the thumb and the index of the other hand and insert them in the circuit. Then exert a pressure on the fingers of the circuit in such a way that they open and that the circuit is thus broken.

It is important to test using a pressure equal to that used by the fingers of the circuit to stay connected together. Likewise, it is important to keep an equal pressure in the fingers of the circuit, without forcing to hold them absolutely together. It is a test of muscular resistance and not of muscular strength.

Then proceed as follows:

1. Ask the question
2. Use the testing fingers (index and thumb) to attempt to break the circuit.
3. If the circuit breaks, that is to say if the fingers of the circuit open like pincers, the answer is YES. If the fingers of the circuit stay firmly connected, the answer is NO.

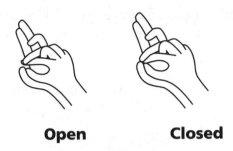

Open   **Closed**

Other Types of Answers

In certain protocols, it is necessary to TEST the quantity (ex.: how many codons, fragments, etc.). In kinesiology, to get an answer, you must ask simple questions leading to a YES or NO answer. Consequently, when searching for a number (how many), you start with a series of questions to determine the order of magnitude, then you work your way toward the exact answer. Here is an example:

Original Question: How many codons does this program contain?

Ask the following questions:

1. *Does the number of codons have 1 number?*   NO
2. *Does the number of codons have 2 numbers?*   NO
3. *Does the number of codons have 3 numbers?*   YES
(We now know that the number of codons is between 100 and 999.)
4. Is the number of codons equal or superior to 500?   NO
(It is therefore a number between 100 and 499.)
5. Is the first digit of the number 1?   NO
6. Is the first digit of the number 2?   YES
The first digit is 2.
7. Is the second number equal or greater than 5?   YES
(It is consequently useless to ask the questions for numbers 0 to 4.)
8. Is the second number 5?   NO
9. Is the second number 6?   NO
10.Is the second number 7?   NO
11.Is the second number 8?   YES
The second number is 8.
12 Is the third number equal or greater than 5?   NO
13.Is the third number 0?   NO
14.Is the third number 1?   YES
The third number is 1.
Answer: There are 281 codons.

You can also find other types of answers by breaking up the original question into a series of questions of the "yes or no" type. Here is a second example:

Original question: Do we need to install a color (answer YES). If yes, **which one?** *To answer the question "which one," draw up a list of colors:*

Question	List of colors	Answer
Is it...	*White*	*NO*
Is it...	*Black*	*NO*
Is it...	*Red*	*NO*
Is it...	*Blue*	*NO*
Is it...	*Green*	*NO*
Is it...	*Orange*	*NO*
Is it...	*Pink*	*NO*
Is it...	*Turquoise*	*NO*
Is it...	*Emerald*	*YES*
	Violet	
	Yellow	
	etc.	

Answer: Emerald

You can also concentrate on each color successively while asking "Is it this color?" until you get a YES.

Even if the fact of asking a series of questions seems a long and fastidious exercise thus explained on paper, in reality, with a little practice, it can be done very quickly.

Appendix III

Possibilities

This appendix constitutes a sort of databank that contains the information to complete the protocols. Test to identify the needed information.

Method:
1. Start by asking the question: "How many items are needed from this appendix?"
2. TEST in which section(s) the data for each item is located by testing the title of each section or its number (1 to 20). Then go to each of the sections that tested YES to test the specific data.

Example: Let us suppose that the answer to Step 1 indicates that you need four items. Then test the title of the 20 sections, which gives:

1	=	NO	
2	=	YES	*hence go to Appendix V, find the mental beliefs, then return to Appendix III to continue testing*
3 and 4	=	NO	
5	=	YES	*in testing the data of section 5, you get "Virus"*
6, 7 and 8	=	NO	
9	=	YES	*in testing the items of section 9, you get "lymph"*
17	=	YES	*the test gives "Earth, pancreas"*

for a total of four inputs.

1. **Emotions:** See Appendix IV.
2. **Mental Beliefs:** See Appendix V.
3. **Spiritual**
    1. Interference – Entities
    2. Chakra – TEST which one (1 to 13) and test to see if it is too open or too closed.
    3. Past life
    4. Astrology/Numerology
    5. Other bodies – TEST which one (1 to 13) and test to see if it needs realignment, if there are holes in the auric field, or other …
    6. Out-of-the-body
    7. Dreams
    8. Stellar
    9. Galactic
    10. Change of frequency
    11. Other
4. **Allergies**
5. **Infections**
    1. Virus
    2. Flu or cold
    3. Chlamydia
    4. Rickettsia
    5. Mycoplasma
    6. Bacteria
    7. Fungus
    8. Parasites
6. **Free radical** (toxins)
    1. Pathological residues
    2. Vaccines
    3. Drugs
    4. Heavy metals
    5. Medication
    6. Radiation
    7. Chemical products
7. **Metabolism**
    1. Assimilation of food – TEST the percentage at which it is accomplished.
    2. Elimination/drainage – TEST the percentage at which it is accomplished.
    3. Digestion – TEST the percentage at which it is accomplished.
    4. Acid/alkaline balance – TEST if too acid or too alkaline.
    5. Blood sugar imbalance
    6. Body fat imbalance
    7. Proteins

8. **Hormonal Imbalance**
    1. Pituitary
    2. Pineal gland
    3. Hypothalamus/thalamus
    4. Thyroid
    5. Thymus
    6. Pancreas
    7. Adrenals
    8. Ovary/Testicles
9. **Circulation**
    1. Blood
    2. Lymph
    3. Nervous influx
    4. Acupuncture (circulation of the meridians)
10. **Structural Problems**
    1. Spine
    2. Skeleton
    3. Organ
    4. Muscles
    5. Ligaments
    6. Fascia
    7. Nerves
    8. DNA
    9. Joints
    10. Other
11. **Teeth**
12. **Chromosome Repair** – See Protocol No. 8.
13. **Colortherapy** –TEST which color the person needs.
14. **Energy Blockage** (i.e. Kundalini, Shushumna, etc.) – (See Appendix VI.)
15. **Genetic Influence**
    1. Dimensions (conception, intra-uterine, present time, etc.)
    2. Miasmas
    3. Transgenerational
    4. Other

16. **Locations** – The different locations of the body have been assembled in five groups, according to the five elements of Chinese medicine. Therefore, test first where the sought data is located, then test which organ in particular.
    1. **FIRE** Element
       1. Heart/circulation
       2. Endocrine glands
       3. Small intestine
    2. **EARTH** Element
       1. Spleen
       2. Pancreas
       3. Stomach/mouth
       4. Nervous system
    3. **METAL** Element
       1. Lungs/nose and sinus
       2. Connective tissue
       3. Colon
       4. Skin
    4. **WATER** Element
       1. Kidneys
       2. Bladder/urethra
       3. Lymph/extracellular or intracellular fluids
       4. Reproductive organs
       5. Ears
    5. **WOOD** Element
       1. Liver
       2. Gall Bladder
       3. Spine and Joints
       4. Eyes
    6. Systems (renal, pulmonary, etc.) – (See Appendix VII.)
    7. Muscles
    8. Brain and nervous system
    9. Acupuncture meridians
17. **Specific Conditions** – A specific condition is a state of the body such as an engorged liver, a cavity filled with coagulated blood, an adherence, an excessive permeability of the small intestine, etc.
18. **Shock** – **TEST** at which age, with whom and under what circumstances.
19. **Other Protocol:** See Table of Contents - Volume I and II
20. **Other**

List of Emotions

Whenever you find the word *emotion* in this appendix, test with this appendix to find which particular emotion is being referred to.

1. A person's name
2. A person's will
3. Abandoned
4. Abnegation
5. Abortion
6. Absent father or mother
7. Absorbed
8. Abused
9. Accomplishment
10. Acts in someone else's stead / replacement
11. Adaptability
12. Addiction to a drug, etc.
13. Adult / program to be able to be accepted
14. Affection is inappropriate
15. Age (Say the age and test if it is accurate.)
16. Aggression
17. Agitation
18. Allergic or auto-immunity in regards to one's own emotions
19. Allergic to an emotion
20. Allergic to parents / children because of their rivalries or demands
21. Altered perceptions
22. Altered psychic perception
23. Always have the same emotional response
24. Ambiguity
25. Angry
26. Another's will
27. Anxiety (thyroid): physical
28. Anxious; adrift because of anxiety
29. Appearance: fear of a good _____, dislikes having a good _____ , to want to avoid attracting attention on a certain part of the body by restraining oneself from having a good _____ , fear/phobia of the jealousy which would cause betrayal if I had a good
30. _____
31. Apprehension
32. Art of selling anything
Artistic expression or all other creation =
33. anxiety and troubles of the nervous system
34. Association, emotions and symptoms
At home / residence (ex.: food = criticism)

1. Aura/nervous system
2. Authority: fear of _____ , to avoid _____ , to need _____ , to take offence at _____ , would like being the _____ .
3. Auto-immunity of the immune system due to an emotion
4. Autosuggestion
5. Bad / vicious
6. Bad perceptions
7. Banished
8. Bearer of an emotion / belief
9. Bearer of an emotion without manifesting it, can bear those of other's or of a society
10. Beauty (personal) = emotion
11. Behaviour and emotion = acts as an infection
12. Being well will make me forget
13. Belief or program that I will hurt myself
14. Belief system and emotion
15. Believes it is irreparable
16. Belligerent
17. Bitterness
18. Blame
19. Blessed future
20. Boredom
21. Brain shock
22. Brainwash
23. Brave
24. Broken (wedding) vows
25. Broken body
26. Broken hearted (how many times)
27. Brother
28. Bulimia
29. Can be manipulated
30. Can give too much support on a psychic level and take another's pain
31. Cannot find
32. Captivity
33. Career
34. Career / profession
35. Central nervous system - memory + emotion
36. Central nervous system and phobia
37. Centered / focused

1. Change
2. Change / to have changed
3. Childhood suffering
4. Choice
5. Choice: to have no ____ , make the wrong ____ , unable to make a ____
6. Circumstances
7. Combat
8. Combined emotion
9. Commitment
10. Commitment: long term
11. Communication
12. Communication: marital
13. Communication: sexual
14. Compassion
15. Compensation and emotions
16. Competition
17. Complacency towards oneself
18. Complain
19. Conflict with a testimony
20. Conflict with humanitarian ideals
21. Conflict with moral standards
22. Confusion
23. Confusion: spiritual
24. Conscience
25. Conservation
26. Conspiracy
27. Contempt
28. Contentment
29. Control
30. Controlling
31. Controlling others
32. Couple problems
33. Courage
34. Cousin
35. Crazy
36. Criminal
37. Cross-link: test with whom? (I am vulnerable to ____ . I am spiritually wed to ____ .)
38. Cyclical reminder
39. Dead: fear of death; fear of someone's death; fear of the death of something (relationship, etc.)
40. Debased
41. Deceitful / lying
42. Defence: no defence or protection
43. Defiance
44. Degeneration of the nervous system because of an emotion
45. Degeneration of the immune system because of an emotion

1. Deprecatory
2. Depression
3. Depression without cause
4. Depression: because of fatigue; because of a broken heart or inherited
5. Depression: suicidal
6. Desire to be controlled
7. Desire to be someone great / good
8. Despairing/desperate
9. Destitute
10. Destroyed
11. Diabolic
12. Dictatorial
13. Difficulty
14. Diminished
15. Disappointed
16. Disappointed: upset
17. Discontent
18. Discontent with oneself
19. Discouragement
20. Discredited
21. Disdain that leads to rage
22. Dishonest
23. Dishonour someone else
24. Dishonoured
25. Disillusioned
26. Disinherited/destitute
27. Dissatisfaction
28. Diversion (ex.: to divert attention from an area of the body…)
29. Divorce
30. Doctor / therapist
31. Dominator
32. Doubt
33. Dreams
34. Ego
35. Embarrassed
36. Emotion about oneself
37. Emotion at a muscular level
38. Emotion due to family
39. Emotion due to relationships
40. Emotion located in a segment of the spine
41. Emotional cerebral fatigue
42. Emotional dependence
43. Emotional desensitization
44. Emotional/spiritual/mental fatigue
45. Emotions: due to miasmas; hereditary
46. Empathy in regards to a situation that we would fix if we could
47. Empathy: spiritual / emotional / physical

1. Encapsulated emotion: find the emotion in question and the location (Appendix III) where it is encapsulated
2. Enlightenment
3. Enthusiasm
4. Envy
5. Established
6. Everybody (thinks …, or is …, etc.)
7. Everybody / the World, etc.
8. Everything is against the person
9. Exaggerated modesty
10. Excessive ego
11. Excuse / symptoms = excuse
12. Expression
13. Expression of one's life
14. Failure (unable to please, inefficient)
15. Failure as a mother / father / sister / brother / spouse / boss / etc.
16. Failure in the eyes of God
17. Failure: professional / social / familial
18. Faith
19. False
20. False personality
21. False prophet
22. Familial
23. Familial cross-link/marriage between cousins
24. Family that vents on him / her
25. Fantasy
26. Father / mother
27. Favouritism in someone else
28. Fear
29. Fear of badly raising one's children
30. Fear of consequences
31. Fear of depending on others
32. Fear of failure: financial, amorous, scholastic, professional, social, etc.
33. Fear of hurting others
34. Fear of receiving
35. Fear of risk
36. Fear of the unknown
37. Fear or phobia of feeling well
38. Fear that an illness will return
39. Fear-stress
40. Feeble emotional power
41. Femininity/masculinity = emotion
42. Financial security towards the future
43. Flashback: scene from the past
44. Flashback: re-enacting the past
45. Foolish
46. For the greater good of…

1. Forced amorous relationships
2. Forgetting oneself
3. Forgiven
4. Forgotten
5. Freedom
6. Friends
7. Friendship
8. Frustration
9. Frustration: sexual
10. Frustration: spiritual
11. Full moon and emotion
12. Furtive / in hiding
13. Future grief
14. Ghost
15. Glory or prestige in being a martyr
16. Goal
17. God
18. Grand-father, grand-mother
19. Guilty
20. Hair
21. Hapless
22. Harmony
23. Hatred: of oneself; of others; of a person in particular
24. Haunted by: — fear; —memory; other
25. Have to / should
26. Have to change / having changed
27. Healing / health
28. Healing: to not heal, to not accept healing, allergic to healing, healing is a stress, non-adaptation to healing, healing = emotion
29. Health problems
30. Hidden emotion (which one?)
31. Hidden rage
32. Hidden rage can lead to being enraged all the time in little doses to avoid losing control
33. Histamine or allergic reaction when thinking of something
34. Hope
35. Hostility
36. Human
37. Humiliated/wounded
38. Hunger
39. Hyperactivity
40. Hypochondriac
41. Hysteria
42. Hysterical
43. I believe I was the cause of…
44. I cannot see / hear / say that I will have or experiment again…
45. I was made to believe that…

1. If it was someone else, what emotion?
2. Ignored
3. Illumination
4. Imagination
5. Imbecile
6. Immature
7. Imminent / menacing
8. Imperious / authoritative
9. Impolite
10. Impossible
11. Impure / foul
12. In mourning
13. Inaccessible
14. Inadequate
15. Inappeasable
16. Incapable
17. Incapable of competing
18. Incapable of creating links
19. Incapable of finding which path to take
20. Incapable of growing
21. Incapable of having fun
22. Incapable of manifesting something of worth in one's life
23. Incapable of trying again
24. Incest: mental; emotional; sexual
25. Incompetent
26. Incomplete ties with the mother / father
27. Indebted towards someone
28. Indomitable
29. Inferiority complex
30. Influenced by others
31. Inhibition
32. Inner child
33. Insecurity / to not feel safe
34. Insensitivity / to be insensitive
35. Insomnia
36. Instable
37. Integrity
38. Interior / exterior stress
39. Internal doubt about things external to oneself
40. Internal reproach
41. Interpretation error
42. Intimidated
43. Intoxication / acclimatization
44. Intrigued by the sordid side of...
45. Introverted
46. Invisible to others' eyes
47. Irresponsible

1. Jealousy
2. Job / employer
3. Joy
4. Knowing one is... + emotion
5. Lack / excess of sexual relations
6. Lack of acceptance
7. Lack of ambition
8. Lack of experience
9. Lack of human warmth
10. Lack of libido
11. Lack of order
12. Lack of peace at an emotional level
13. Lack of physical contact
14. Lack of sympathy / compassion
15. Lead others down the wrong path
16. Legitimate defence / instinct to
17. Lies
18. Life
19. Life and emotion
20. Life failure
21. Lifestyle
22. Linked by vows (may be wedding vows)
23. Linked or joined to another
24. Little or not loved
25. Lost
26. Love of oneself, of another
27. Love = emotion (test which one).
28. Love that is altered / mutated when someone has lived with a person which was always on the brink of a nervous breakdown but who never really had one
29. Love that is not reciprocated
30. Macho
31. Maniac-depressive
32. Manipulator
33. Manner of conceiving of a situation
34. Many people
35. Marginal personality
36. Marriage
37. Meditation
38. Melancholy
39. Memory
40. Miscarriage
41. Missing twin (intrauterine)
42. Money
43. Morbid thoughts
44. Morose
45. Mortal / dead
46. Mothering (to have lacked...)
47. Mothering (to need...) – or be nurtured

1. Motivation: intrinsic; extrinsic
2. Movement or travelling that triggers memories
3. Multiple personalities
4. Must repent for something
5. Mysterious / supernatural
6. Narcissism
7. Need affection
8. Need amnesia
9. Need escape
10. Need freedom
11. Need love / to want to love
12. Need more attention
13. Need more pleasure
14. Need recognition
15. Need support
16. Need to abandon oneself to a problem
17. Need to be cherished
18. Need to be framed
19. Need to be guided
20. Need to be loved unconditionally
21. Need to be punished by God
22. Need to cherish
23. Need to fix things
24. Need to forgive
25. Need to have children
26. Need to have someone else punish us
27. Need to prove something
28. Need to punish oneself
29. Need to suffer
30. Nervous breakdown: of the digestive system; of the physical body; pelvic; familial / inherited; intra-uterine; postpartum; liver / thyroid; auric; another's
31. Nervous/unable to relax
32. Nervousness
33. New decor
34. Nitpicker/quibbler
35. No blessed future
36. No future
37. No peace of the spirit
38. No right to live
39. Non-perception of an emotion
40. Not blessed
41. Not complementary
42. Not finished
43. Not well adjusted
44. Nutritional disorder: bulimia, anorexia
45. Obligation
46. Obsession

1. Offensive in public
2. On the defensive
3. One must not speak of it
4. One who speaks ill of others / denouncer
5. One's own intent
6. Oneself
7. Opinion
8. Opportunity
9. Oppression
10. Organization
11. Other
12. Outrageously generous
13. Pain: emotional, physical, spiritual, mental
14. Panic – confusion
15. Paranoia: in general; towards someone; towards something
16. Passive-aggressive
17. Past-related sorrow
18. Paternity / maternity
19. Peace
20. People aren't interested in me / neglected
21. Perfectionist
22. Persecuted
23. Persecution
24. Personal value: allergic to one's ____ ; to lack ____ (can be ingrained)
25. Perturbed
26. Pessimistic
27. Phobia and emotion
28. Phobia of being a champion or of being important
29. Phobia of rage
30. Phobia: — of hurting oneself, — of hospitals, etc.
31. Phobias
32. Physical abuse
33. Physical illness
34. Pleasure / fun
35. Point of view
36. Poor example
37. Poor me
38. Positive thinking hides an emotion
39. Positivity (inversed or negated)
40. Possessive
41. Post-shock, post-traumatic syndrome
42. Premonition
43. Problem – his/hers or someone else's
44. Program that has been erased
45. Programmed to accept children
46. Projection

1. Protection
2. Protective screen
3. Psychological abuse
4. Psychosis
5. Public
6. Rage
7. Rage / repressed hatred
8. Rage combined with hatred
9. Rage transformed into another emotion
10. Rape / trauma
11. Rape: physical; psychological; of the residence; or any encroachment of privacy or intimacy
12. Reality
13. Rebellion
14. Recognize one's femininity / masculinity
15. Recompense
16. Recurring thoughts
17. Rejected by the family
18. Relationships
19. Relationships: amorous; friendly; professional; social; etc.
20. Remorse (to have done too much)
21. Resentful
22. Resentment
23. Resistance to healing
24. Resistance to something – like being helped
25. Respect (make a sentence with this word)
26. Responsibility of having a family
27. Retirement
28. Revenge (hatred)
29. Rigid/intransigent
30. Sad
31. Satisfied
32. Saving oneself
33. Scapegoat
34. Sceptic
35. Schizophrenia
36. Self-criticism
37. Self-destruction/ suicide
38. Self-doubt
39. Self-esteem
40. Selfish / bossy
41. Self-perception
42. Self-punishment
43. Self-rejection
44. Self-revenge
45. Sexual abuse (molestation /vicious)
46. Sexual fantasy
47. Sexual trauma (rape)
48. Shaken

1. Shame
2. Shock
3. Shock related to emotional healing
4. Should not
5. Sister
6. Sitting on the fence
7. Small size / big size
8. Someone else's emotion (which one/whose?)
9. Someone else's intent
10. Someone is venting on him/her
11. Son/daughter
12. Sorry
13. Special occasion
14. Spiritual wound
15. Starved (spiritual or emotional)
16. Stature
17. Stolen
18. Strength
19. Stress + emotion
20. Stress and non-perception
21. Stress caused by a phobia
22. Stress comes from: — inherited; — intra-uterine; — birth, — conception; miasmas (find the number of generations); — the chromosome level
23. Stress due to an interpretation error (ex.: love = manipulation)
24. Stress due to bereavement
25. Stress of someone who struggles in life
26. Stress related to nerves
27. Stress related to one's death
28. Stress: fear of ____; phobia of ____; to be used to ____
29. Stress: unable to release stress
30. Stricken
31. Stubborn
32. Stupid
33. Success (to not be programmed for...)
34. Suffering
35. Superficial emotion
36. Suppressed emotion
37. Survival
38. Suspicions
39. Sympathy
40. Symptoms, emotion
41. Take care of..., fear of not being cared for; to need to be loved unconditionally; being strong = to not receive warmth anymore; fear of feeling that someone is taking care of us; fear of being led on the wrong path because of our need to be fed by someone else

1. Talent
2. Tears
3. Terror
4. The body believes it is a man / woman
5. The body is unable to heal completely, can only survive, undoing all of the healing or positive emotion, because of the fear of failure
6. The core emotion / first emotion
7. The mistake of one's life
8. Thief
9. Thin / fat
10. Thwarted
11. Timid – fear of success
12. To abandon
13. To act according to one's convictions
14. To act like
15. To allow
16. To allow one: to hurt oneself; to fail, etc.
17. To avoid a subject, an emotion
18. To be a champion
19. To be a student / to learn
20. To be abandoned
21. To be adopted
22. To be afraid
23. To be afraid one's children will turn badly
24. To be allergic to responsibility
25. To be alone
26. To be an example
27. To be attached, tied
28. To be bad
29. To be belittled
30. To be blamed
31. To be blond, brown, auburn, etc.
32. To be conscious
33. To be deprived of
34. To be deserted/abandoned
35. To be doubted by someone
36. To be emotionally strong
37. To be good
38. To be in bad company
39. To be known for
40. To be left for dead
41. To be livid
42. To be manipulated or to want to be…
43. To be needy
44. To be nice
45. To be on bad terms with someone
46. To be oneself, natural
47. To be open to…

1. To be programmed
2. To be punished
3. To be pushed away
4. To be rebuffed
5. To be responsible for
6. To be restrained by
7. To be seen as someone else
8. To be sorrowful
9. To be supposed to…
10. To be torn between two: people, situation
11. To be unable to do something
12. To be unable to do something: frustration
13. To be unable to eliminate an emotion
14. To be unable to find something
15. To be unappreciated
16. To be undesired
17. To be undiscovered
18. To be unrecognized
19. To believe a falsehood
20. To believe falsehoods about oneself
21. To belong to each other
22. To blame oneself
23. To choose the wrong path / direction in one's life
24. To confiscate
25. To conspire
26. To convalesce / healing
27. To create
28. To create one's own future: financial or other (which one?)
29. To denigrate
30. To depend on another to feel good about oneself
31. To depend on someone for one's self-esteem
32. To desire a symptom or something negative
33. To destroy a part of oneself
34. To disobey
35. To dominate oneself
36. To express ones emotions or opinions = emotion
37. To faint
38. To falsify
39. To feel attacked
40. To feel betrayed
41. To feel broken
42. To feel creative about the future
43. To feel criticized
44. To feel cut off from the world
45. To feel dominated / controlled
46. To feel empty

1. To feel empty of all positive emotion
2. To feel indebted towards someone
3. To feel isolated
4. To feel less than…
5. To feel poor or to be poor
6. To feel proud of oneself
7. To feel rejected
8. To feel separated from…
9. To feel that someone needs us
10. To feel that we are being lacked respect
11. To feel threatened
12. To feel thwarted
13. To feel tired of…
14. To feel used
15. To forgive: – oneself, – others, – God, – one's family, etc.
16. To give but not to receive
17. To give the example
18. To go bankrupt
19. To have an opinion / a judgment
20. To have been beaten / to be physically or mentally beaten
21. To have been neglected
22. To have a clear conscience
23. To have committed a crime
24. To have done a disservice to one's family
25. To have given a bad performance
26. To have lacked physical contact in one's childhood
27. To have lost control
28. To have lost everything
29. To have lost one's life
30. To have lost the desire to …
31. To have lost the desire to live
32. To have lost the taste for life
33. To have made a mistake
34. To have no need of someone
35. To have no voice
36. To have not been accepted as a child
37. To have not established good parental ties with one's children
38. To have not received familial benediction
39. To have resentment
40. To have value
41. To have zero emotion
42. To lack confidence in myself; hence to defend myself from something bad for me
43. To lack conscience of oneself or degenerate perception of one's sense of self
44. To lack desire

1. To lack emotions
2. To lack freedom
3. To lack goals / objectives
4. To lack respect
5. To lack the right to a prosperous / happy / … future
6. To lack the right to feel good
7. To lack the right to love
8. To lack the right to or to not find one's…
9. To lack the right to say or repeat
10. To lack trust in one's words
11. To lack value
12. To lack work
13. To leave
14. To let go of someone dear to us
15. To lie
16. To lose face
17. To lose faith
18. To lose one's cool
19. To lower oneself
20. To make love = an emotion
21. To make plans for the future
22. To miss someone terribly
23. To misunderstand someone's body language
24. To move
25. To neglect
26. To not believe in God
27. To not belong to oneself
28. To not feel capable of
29. To not feel one has a right to love
30. To not feel safe
31. To not feel useful
32. To not have what one wants
33. To not know what / which to choose
34. To not know what one wants
35. To not know where to place oneself / live
36. To not permit oneself to: heal; be loved; etc.
37. To not want to be different / special
38. To not want to be normal
39. To not worry / to be carefree
40. To nurture / to take care of…
41. To pretend
42. To prevent oneself from crying
43. To program oneself to die young
44. To protect oneself (question of survival)
45. To react (ex. to others' stress)
46. To remember – to not want to remember
47. To remember a forgotten grief
48. To repeat the same things over and over
49. To retire / give up

1. To ruin
2. To ruminate about a thought, an action, an idea
3. To run away / to flee
4. To sabotage
5. To speak of = emotion
6. To struggle for survival or difficulty to make ends meet
7. To take someone else's emotions on oneself
8. To think of others before oneself
9. To trust
10. To unhook
11. To wish for someone to die
12. To wish to die
13. To love the attention that comes with violence, abuse, attack, contradiction, suffering, etc.
14. Tortured or need to be tortured
15. Tragedy
16. Troubled
17. Truth
18. Unaccepted
19. Unaccomplished / without talents
20. Unassailable
21. Unattached / free
22. Unavowable (crime)
23. Unbalanced interpretation
24. Uncertain
25. Uncle / aunt
26. Unconscious
27. Undecided
28. Unfaithful
29. Unhappy
30. Unmasked
31. Unresolved situation
32. Unsupported
33. Unvanquished
34. Unworthy
35. Useless
36. Value system and emotion
37. Victim
38. Victim and emotion
39. Victim of others' symptoms, of their illnesses, emotions or inherited traits
40. Vindictive
41. Violence
42. Visualization: incapable of doing a ... ; ... excessive
43. Vocation
44. Voluntary debasement

1. Vows (maybe wedding vows)
2. Vulnerable
3. Waiting for oneself
4. Waiting for others
5. Waiting for something: expectations
6. Want to be loved
7. Want to be protected
8. Want to be someone else
9. Want to devour food / sugar
10. Way of thinking – inherited?
11. Weakness
12. Wealth
13. When one uses a negative emotion for…
14. Where is my place?
15. Which emotion do I need to solve this problem?
16. Who doubts
17. Who doubts God
18. Wisdom
19. Without affection
20. Without end / never
21. Without hope
22. Without pity
23. Without recourse
24. Without remorse
25. Words
26. Work
27. Worried
28. Worry
29. Wrinkled
30. Wrong direction in life
31. Wrong sex

Emotions and Affirmations (Intents) for the Mental Aspect

Vulnerability / Wound	New Structure
1. Fear	*I am safe.*
2. Wounds	*I am free.*
3. Vengeance	*I am at peace.*
4. Does not accept oneself	*I accept myself.*
5. Anger	*I take care of others and myself.*
6. Friction – family	*I am both wanted and loved.*
7. Rejection	*I am perfect.*
8. Sexual guilt	*I am love and sexuality.*
9. Loss of power	*The world and I are safe.*
10. No direction	*I go forward in life with ease.*
11. Self-hatred	*I am filled with joy and love for myself.*
12. To hold on to guilt	*I let the past go, I am free, I forgive myself.*
13. Not trusting	*I trust in life, I am safe.*
1. Judgement	*My feelings are normal and without risk.*
2. Narrow mindedness	*I am completely open-minded.*
3. Suppression	*I take charge of my life.*
4. Scattered	*I center myself.*
5. Tension	*I trust in life, I am safe.*
6. Anxious	*It is joy that I welcome.*
7. Lack of joy	*I have new joyous ideas.*
8. Resistance	*I go with the flow, lightly.*
9. Defeat	*I choose to live my life now even if I have made mistakes in the past.*
10. Stubborn	*My whole life is in change.*
11. Overprotective of others	*I am free to be myself.*
12. Overprotection	*I can grow without risk.*

Vulnerability / Wound	New Structure
1. Failure	*I am adequate at all times.*
2. Resentment	*I let the past go.*
3. Sadness	*I fill my world with joy.*
4. Hatred	*I forgive all my past experiences.*
5. Feeling trapped	*I travel through time and space with ease.*
6. Childhood pain	*I forgive the entire world.*
7. Feeling alone	*I am safe, all is well.*
1. Hypersensitive	*I am always safe and sheltered.*
2. Stifled	*I express myself with ease.*
3. Sad	*Joy, joy, joy flows in my body and in my head.*
4. Isolated	*I am one with everything.*
5. Worry	*I want to let go with joy.*
6. Bitterness	*Life is sweet and so am I.*
7. Uncertainty	*I love myself and approve of myself.*
8. Heaviness	*There is time and space for all that I do.*
9. Disappointment	*I fulfill myself.*
10. Exhaustion	*My life is easy and joyful.*
11. Remorse	*I am at peace where I am.*
1. Frustration	*I transform all types of criticisms.*
2. Shame	*Every experience brings only good.*
3. Without honor	*I am flexible and malleable.*
4. To justify or justifying	*I search for love and find it everywhere.*
5. Depression	*I love life to the extreme.*
6. Jealousy	*There is enough for everyone.*
7. Undecided	*My decisions are always perfect for me.*
8. Worrying	*I am marvellous and I support myself.*
9. Easily critical	*I am going towards my greater good.*
10. Hopeless	*My life improves from day to day.*
11. Insecurity	*I am free to speak in my name.*
12. To feel attacked	*I am safe and sheltered at all times.*

Vulnerability / Wound	New Structure
1. Without support	*Life supports all my thoughts.*
2. Inflexibility	*I am open to new ideas.*
3. Without courage	*I know life is in my favour.*
4. Obstinate	*It is safe to consider other points of view.*
5. Obsessions	*I trust in the process of life.*
6. Undecided	*I take decisions easily.*
7. Humiliation	*I surpass all my limits.*
8. Selfish	*I create a safe world in which to live.*
9. Persecution	*I see life in an eternal and joyous manner.*
10. Denial	*I take pleasure in all that I am.*
11. Confusion	*My mind is relaxed and at peace.*
12. Irritation	*All is peaceful.*
13. Defeat	*I choose to be a winner in life.*
14. Worry	*I choose to have a blessed future in regards to …*

Appendix VI

Psychic Energy Blockages

1. *SUSHUMNA* – Energy canal through which the Kundalini flows and which corresponds to the spinal chord of the physical body.

2. *IDA* and *PINGALA* – Vibrational canals located to the left (*Ida*) and right (*Pingala*) of the *Sushumna*. Ida and Pingala are considered to be energy nerves (being therefore part of the nervous system of the vibrational body) located on each side of the *Sushumna*. They end at the nose after having travelled through the back of the head.

3. *KUNDALINI* – Latent energy which, once awakened, rises in the canal of the *Sushumna*. This phenomenon, called "rise of the *Kundalini*", can lead to illumination.

4. *PRANA* – Molecule of subtle energy inhaled in the air that feeds the etherical bodies. Its role for the etherical bodies is akin to that of oxygen for the physical body.

5. *CONNECTION* of the *IDA* and the *PINGALA* – **TEST** the connection at the level of the base chakra.

6. *VITAL ENERGY* – Life force: that which keeps us alive.

7. *PRANA* / **DEAD VITAL ENERGY**

8. *PRANA* / **VITAL ENERGY STOLEN BY ANOTHER**

9. *SOUL* – PARENTAL SOUL

10. **ETHERIC CORDS BETWEEN THE PERSON AND SOMEONE ELSE:**
    A. TEST with whom;
    B. TEST in which chakra(s);
    C. TEST in which direction: from the other to the person or the opposite;
    D. TEST if it is necessary to undo the connection and reconnect the cord in the heart chakra or if it is necessary to degenerate the cord (most often, if the other person is dead).

11. **DEAD ENERGY**

12. **LOCATION (Appendix III, No. 16) + BLOCKED ENERGY**

13. **WOUND** – TEST if it is mental, spiritual, physical, emotional, chemical or other.

14. **COSMIC GRID**

15. **POISOINING, TOXICITY, ALLERGIES, SHOCK or ACUTE DEATH SYNDROME in the CHAKRAS, the ETHERIC BODIES or other non-physical locations.**

16. **COSMIC ORBIT** – TEST if it is broken or blocked by evaluating its circuit: in front, from the kidneys to the perineum, by ascending the length of the back up to the head, then once more in front, by descending towards the navel.

17. *MERKABAH* – (See Appendix I.) There are three fields superposed on one another around our body: physical, mental and emotional. If these fields are turned by connecting the mental, the emotional and the physical body, then the mental field turns towards the left, the emotional towards the right and the physical remains immobile. When these fields turn at a very precise speed and in a specific way, it may create a sphere.

18. **PATHOLOGY OF THE CHAKRAS** (1 to 13 chakras)
    A. Disinsertion;
    B. Pathological insertion: TEST
       (i)   if there is splitting;
       (ii)   if it is at the wrong location in the body;
       (iii)   if the rotation is in the right direction (ex.: backwards);
    C. Well inserted, but a change in the rotational axis (especially the 1st chakra);
    D. Vibration rate too high or too low;
    E. Other.

19. **PATHOLOGY OF ETHERIC BODIES** – TEST which one(s) – a count of about 7, sometimes more. Also TEST:
    A. If there is dissociation;
    B. If there is a hole, a tear or a stain (black or gray);
    C. If there is a transfer of consciousness in another dimension, another reality or another orbit (ex.: mental illness);
    D. If the person is stuck in no-time or no-space;
    E. If the person is stuck in a polarity through time, space, the universes, etc.

20. **SOUND**
    a) TEST if a specific sound is missing from the voice of the person when speaking of the past, the present or the future.

Chakra	Sound	Mantra	Music
1st	do	lam	strong/rhythmical
2nd	re	vam	light
3rd	mi	ram	fire rhythms
4th	fa	yam	new age
5th	so	ham	harmonic
6th	la	ksham	of the Spheres
7th	si (ti)	ohm	silence

    b) TEST if a vowel is missing in the voice of the person when speaking of the past, present or future. If YES, TEST which one: a, e, i, o, u.

21. **SHAMANIC** – TEST:
    A. if there are body parts that are missing or lost;
    B. if the soul is disjoined;
    C. if there is a distortion of an energetic shamanic site.

22. **VIBRATIONAL FREQUENCY IN HERTZ** (0 to 78) – TEST:
    A. at which frequency is the body vibrating?
    B. what is the best frequency for the body?

23. **CONNECTION AND ALIGNMENT WITH THE CENTER OF THE EARTH** – TEST at which percentage the person is connected to the center of the Earth.

24. **PLANETS** – Earth, Sun, Moon, Mercury, Venus, Mars, Jupiter, Saturn, Uranus, Neptune, Pluto, Chiron, Asteroids, other.

25. **SERIES OF NUMBERS / NUMEROLOGY** – TEST which number(s).

26. **TIMELINES** – TEST:
    A. on how many timelines the person is living;
    B. how many themes crisscross;
    C. how many points they have in common.

27. **HOLOGRAM OR DISTORTION OF REALITY** – TEST:
    A. if the person is conscious of it and able to degenerate it. If NO, TEST why by using Appendixes III, IV, V and VI;
    B. if it blocks access to the program of self-love.

28. *MUDRAS* – The *mudras* are hand positions that help produce psychic energy and channel *prana* in a precise direction.
    TEST each *mudra* by joining your fingertips in the following manner:
    A. thumb and index finger;
    B. thumb and middle finger;
    C. thumb and ring finger;
    D. thumb and pinky;
    E. thumb and index + middle fingers;
    For each position, TEST if the *mudra* is too open, too closed or blocked.

29. **DIMENSIONS** – There can be more than 12 dimensions. TEST:
    A. the connection to each dimension;
    B. the stabilization;
    C. the realignment.

30. **GEOMETRY** – TEST if the body of the person or its environment needs a specific geometric symbol: Reiki, spiral, triangle, square, circle, infinity symbol, lightning symbol, sphere, tetrahedron, hexahedron, octahedron, icosahedron, dodecahedron, octahedral cube, rhombic dodecahedron, metatron cube, tree of life, flower of life, fruit of life, icosahedric starred dodecahedron, runic symbol, other.

31. **OTHER**

List of Systems

1. Mitochondrial genetic system
2. Haemopoietic system
3. Chamber system
4. Emotional system
5. Cell elimination system
6. Electromagnetic system
7. Integumentary system
8. Peripheral nervous system
9. Urogenital system
10. Lymphatic system
11. Reticuloendothelial system
12. Pelvic system
13. Solar plexus
14. Gastrointestinal system
15. Digestive valve system
16. ATP/ADP system *(glucose + proteins)*
17. Dermatological system
18. Detoxification system
19. Cerebral vascular system
20. Metabolic system
21. Respiratory system
22. Immune system
23. Diaphragmatic system
24. Exteroceptive system

1. Cardiovascular system
2. Circulation + system
3. Celiac plexus
4. Interstitial system
5. Sense organ system: *ear, eye, nose, muscle and tongue*
6. Teeth system
7. Vision system
8. Hearing system
9. Vestibular system *(auditory pathways)*
10. Respiratory system
11. Cranial system
12. Psychic system
13. Central nervous system
14. DNA system
15. Endocrine system
16. Sinus system
17. Sensory system
18. Muscular system
19. Skeletal system
20. Smooth muscle system + the specific system ; *ex.: smooth muscle + digestive system*
21. Excretory system
22. All systems

Appendix VIII

Selected Readings

Anand, Margo. Illustrated by Atma Priti, *The Art of Sexual Magic*. USA: Putnam Books, 1989.

Anand, Margot. *The Art of Everyday Ecstasy*. Bantam, 1999.

Braden, Gregg. *Walking Between Worlds: The Science of Compassion*. USA: Sacred Spaces Ancient Wisdom, 1997.

Braden, Gregg, *Awakening to Zero Point*. USA: LL Productions.

Braden, Gregg, *The Isaiah Effect: Decoding the Lost Science of Prayer and Prophecy*. USA: Crown, 2000.

Carroll, Lee and Tober, Jan. *The Indigo Children: The New Kids Have Arrived*. USA: Hay House, 1999.

Carroll, Lee. Kryon - *The End Times (Kryon Writings; 1), New Information for Personal Peace*, 1993.

Chia, Mantak and Chia, Maneewan. *Healing Love through the Tao - Cultivating Female Sexual Energy*. USA: Healing Tao Books, 1993.

Chia, Mantak and Winn, Michael. *Taoist Secrets of Love - Cultivating Male Sexual Energy*. USA: Aurora Press, 1983.

Clow, Barbara Hand. *The Pleiadian Agenda - A New Cosmology for the Age of Light*. Bear and Company, 1995.

DeRohan, Ceanne. *The Right Use of Will*. Sante Fe, N.M.: Four Winds Publications 1986.

Diamond, John. *Your Body Doesn't Lie: A New Simple Test Measures Impacts Upon Your Life Energy*. New York: Warner Books, Inc., 1983.

Frissell, Bob. *Nothing in this Book Is True, but It's Exactly How Things Are*. USA: Frog, 1994.

Frissell, Bob. *Something in This Book Is True*. USA: Frog Ltd., 2003.

Frissell, Bob. *You Are a Spiritual Being Having a Human Experience*. USA: Frog Ltd., 2000.

Icke, David. *The Biggest Secret*. USA: Bridge of Love Publication, 1999-2002.

Katz, Pamela K., Tobin, Jacqueline L. and Cheng, Shi-Huei (Illustrator). *The Tao of Women*, 1995-06.

Kauffman, Barry, *Happiness is a choice*, 1994.

Lanctot, Ghyslaine. *The Medical Mafia*. Quebec: Here's the Key, 1995.

Manning, Jeane and Begich, Dr. Nick. *Angels Don't Play this Haarp, Advances in Tesla Technology* (HAARP: High-frequency Active Auroral Research Project), 1995.

Marciniak, Barbara. Edited by Tera Thomas, *Bringers of the Dawn, Teachings from the Pleiadians*. USA: Bear & Co., 1992.

Marciniak, Barbara with Marciniak, Karen and Thomas, Tera, *Earth, Pleiadian Keys to the Living Library*. USA: Bear & Co., 1995.

Marciniak, Barbara. *Family of Light, Pleiadian Tales & Lessons in Living*. USA: Bear & Co., 1999.

Melchizedek, Drunvalo. *The Ancient Secret of the Flower of Life - Volume 1*. USA: Light Technology Publishing, 1998.

Melchizedek, Drunvalo. *The Ancient Secret of the Flower of Life - Volume 2*. USA: Light Technology Publishing, 2000.

Myss, Caroline. *Anatomy of the Spirit, The Seven Stages of Power and Healing*. USA: Three Rivers Press, 1996.

Myss, Caroline. *Why People Don't Heal and How They Can*. The Crown Publishing Group, 1997.

Orloff, Judith. *Second Sight - A Psychiatrist Clairvoyant Tells her Extraordinary Story and Shows You How to Discover Your Psychic Gifts*. USA: Warner, 1997.

Page, Linda. *Healthy Healing, 11th edition*. USA: Healthy Healing, 1997.

Pearl, Eric. *The Reconnection: Heal Others, Heal Yourself*. USA: Hay House, 2003.

Pert, Candace B. *Molecules of Emotion, Why You Feel the Way You Feel*. USA: Simon & Schuster, A Touchstone Book, 1997.

Schulz, Mona Lisa. *Awakening Intuition, Using Your Mind-Body Network for Insight and Healing*. USA, Three River Press, 2002.

Tansley, David V. *Chakras-Rays and Radionics*. England: C.W. Daniel, 1984.

Tansley, David V. in collaboration with Malcolm Rae and Dr. Aubrey T. Westlake. *Dimensions of Radionics, Techniques of Instrumented Distant-Healing - A Manual of Radionic Theory and Practice*, 1977, 1992.

Wolinsky, Stephen. *The Dark Side of the Inner Child*. USA: Bramble Co., 1993.

Wolinsky, Stephen and Ryan, Margaret O. *Trances People Live, Healing Approaches in Quantum Psychology*. USA: Bramble Co., 1991.

Wright, Machaelle Small. *Behaving as if the God in All Life Mattered*. USA: Perelandra, 1987.

SUGGESTED WEB SITE on the Russian study mentioned on page 52:

Garjajev, Pjootr (biologist). Russian Studies on DNA, www.forsarbludorf.com., Vernetzte Intelligenz, Von Grazyna and Vranx Bludorf, ISBN 3930233237.

Appendix IX

Biography and Courses

Biography

Professionally trained in naturopathy, Kishori Aird is currently a medical-intuitive practitioner. All medical-intuitive doctors have their own methods of reading symptoms and re-establishing the vital current after identifying blockages. Ms. Aird is no different; she uses, among other methods, *Reprogramming Kinesiology.*

The path to medical intuition is taken more often nowadays than it was ten years ago. Ms. Aird has been on a long, spiritual and alternative journey. She lived in an ashram when she was 18. At 20, she took courses in nursing to become a midwife. At 25, after once again living in an ashram for two years, she started a family and moved to Ottawa where she worked at the L'Arche de Jean Vanier (home for people with developmental disabilities). In 1986, she returned to Montreal and started taking new courses in healing with crystals and hypnotherapy. Since the Harmonic Convergence in 1987, she completed therapeutic training based on naturopathy and emotional therapies. She is trained in Tantra and is a Reiki Master.

In 1990, she was introduced to reprogramming kinesiology on the American West Coast and had the opportunity to work in a renowned chiropractic and naturopathic clinic. In 1993, after this period of training in the field of naturopathy and kinesiology, she opened her own clinic and started working with clients by telephone as a professional in medical intuition. Since 1994, she has been giving courses on how to use kinesiology, DNA reprogramming and the art of developing one's own medical intuition.

In the summer of 1997, she began studies on DNA and the methods for reprogramming and reclaiming ownership of our DNA. She then went on to develop the reprogramming techniques that she teaches today.

Courses

Kishori Aird teaches the reprogramming protocols found in *DNA Demystified* (Volume I) and *DNA and Quantum Choices* (Volume II). In these courses, she introduces the protocols and teaches students how to make new connections and reprogram themselves using medical intuition.

For your information, you should know that there are no teachers currently authorized by Kishori Institute to teach the content of these books. To protect yourself, please consult us before registering for a training session on DNA Reprogramming. At this time, only Kishori Institute offers training courses.

For more information on training, please contact the Kishori Institute, Inc.

P.O. Box 252, Magog, JIX 3W8
Tel.: (819) 868-1284, Fax: (819) 868-9007
Web site: www. Kishori.org

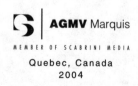

MEMBER OF SCABRINI MEDIA

Quebec, Canada
2004